PSYCHOLOGY AND PSYCHIATRY FOR NURSES

Fourth Edition

PSYCHOLOGY AND PSYCHIATRY FOR NURSES

FOURTH EDITION

Peter Dally M.B., F.R.C.P., F.R.C.Psych., D.P.M.
Department of Psychological Medicine, Westminster Hospital, London

Heather Harrington S.R.N., R.M.N.
Queen Mary's Hospital, London

THE ENGLISH UNIVERSITIES PRESS LIMITED

ISBN 0340 190647 Paper Edition
ISBN 0 3 40 190655 Boards Edition

First printed 1964
Second edition 1967
Reprinted (with corrections) 1969
Third edition 1972
Reprinted 1973, 1974
Fourth edition 1975

The English Universities Press Ltd
St Paul's House Warwick Lane
London EC4P 4AH

Text set in 11pt Monotype Ehrhardt,
printed by letterpress, and bound in
Great Britain at The Pitman Press, Bath

Introduction

Psychology is the study and understanding of *normal* mental functions and behaviour. *Psychiatry*, on the other hand, is concerned with the study and treatment of disordered mental processes.

Great changes have occurred during the past twenty years in psychiatry. Powerful new drugs, which influence mental states and behaviour, have become available. Medical and public attitudes to psychiatric disorders have changed. The Mental Health Act of 1959 recognizes that psychiatry is a branch of medicine and that, like any other illness, mental disorders require treatment. Any mentally ill patient can now be admitted to any hospital for treatment. As a result, nurses in general hospitals encounter more and more patients with psychiatric illnesses. Nurses trained in mental illness now find themselves working in units attached to general hospitals.

In addition, the importance of psychological factors in organic illness, and their influence on the behaviour of both patients and nursing staff, have been increasingly realized. All nurses are now expected to have some understanding of psychology in order to appreciate these problems.

We have written this book both for nurses in general training and those training as mental nurses. Part One concerns psychology and its influence in general hospitals. Part Two deals with psychiatry, and the management and treatment of psychiatric patients.

We have included a *glossary* at the end of Part Two.

Editors' Foreword

The scope of this series has increased since it was first established, and it now serves a wide range of medical, nursing and ancillary professions, in line with the present trend towards the belief that all who care for patients in a clinical context have an increasing amount in common.

The texts are carefully prepared and organized so that they may be readily kept up to date as the rapid developments of medical science demand. The series already includes many popular books on various aspects of medical and nursing care, and reflects the increased emphasis on community care.

The increasing specialization in the medical profession is fully appreciated and the books are often written by Physicians or Surgeons in conjunction with specialist nurses. For this reason, they will not only cover the syllabus of training of the General Nursing Council, but will be designed to meet the needs of those undertaking trainings controlled by the Joint Board of Clinical Studies set up in 1970.

Contents

PART ONE

Psychology

I

EVOLUTION AND ADAPTATION

All life must adapt to its surroundings. Adaptation to the external environment is necessary for survival.

An independent single living cell, such as an amoeba, must continually search for food, escape from enemies, avoid drying up and remain within certain limits of temperature in order to survive.

Life began with single living cells, in direct contact with their surroundings. Gradually organisms evolved and were composed of many cells, increasingly separated from the exterior. A nervous system developed and allowed communication and co-ordination between different parts of the body. As organisms became more complex, so did the nervous system. It enabled the animal to perceive changes in both the external and the internal environment, and react appropriately to changing events in both. The internal environment of the highly developed organism is much more complicated than the internal environment of a single cell. Not only are there many cells of many different types but there are also body fluids which bathe these cells continuously.

The fact that man has a highly developed internal environment allows him to be free of many of the restrictions of the external environment which limit simpler organisms. Man is able to be mobile. We can live at the North Pole or the Equator and in dry or wet regions. But it is vitally important for our bodies that the internal environment shall remain steady. The constancy of the internal environment is called *homeostasis*.

Any change is immediately corrected by sensitive mechanisms in the body which act through the nervous system by *reflex action*. Thus, for instance, a fall in blood pressure is corrected by an increased heart rate and a constriction of blood vessels running to the less important structures, such as the skin. This is why a patient suffering from shock is pale. Such changes occur reflexly, and often without our being aware of them.

Although we are now less dependent on the external environment than were our primitive ancestors we still have to obtain food and avoid enemies. In addition a partner has to be found for sexual reproduction. Simple reflex behaviour, although suitable for adjusting the internal environment, is now altogether too crude and unadaptable for dealing with the external environment.

3

At a certain stage in the evolution of organisms, *instincts* developed, and they reached their peak in the insect world. Instincts are unlearned inherited forms of behaviour, particularly concerned with self-preservation and reproduction. Many insects perform the most complicated pattern of behaviour, which is common to the whole species, and cannot be altered by experience. They seem to be fixed and innate. At this level of evolutionary development, such behaviour is unadaptable. But as the evolutionary ladder is ascended, instinctive behaviour becomes increasingly adaptable and liable to be modified by experience. This tendency reaches its maximum in man, and the human infant is born with few established or fixed patterns of behaviour. A baby can breathe, suck, swallow and perform other actions necessary for life, but in most other respects he is totally dependent on adults for his wants.

It is because of his immature and underdeveloped state at birth and his long dependence on adults that man has become so flexible. At birth his central nervous system is still relatively underdeveloped, and it is capable of being moulded in many directions by environmental pressures throughout childhood and perhaps later to a lesser extent. Family and social differences will direct his outlook and influence his behaviour. He still has need for sex, food and other biological necessities, for fundamentally he remains an animal. But the way he satisfies these needs will depend on patterns of behaviour formed in his nervous system during his early years. It is better therefore to speak of human *needs* rather than of human *instincts*.

An infant's needs—for example hunger—cause him to feel tense and uncomfortable; he then cries and behaves characteristically. Satisfaction following feeding produces pleasure and relaxation. Feelings of pleasure, or 'unpleasure', are known as *emotions* and are probably the only emotions a newborn infant has. But as the brain matures, new and derived emotions develop. Emotions provide much of the drive behind our behaviour.

Intelligence, which depends on the development of the cerebral cortex, is the main means by which man is able to adapt to his environment. But natural forces—food, warmth, safety and so on—are no longer the most serious problems for most of us. We also have to adapt to the demands and restrictions of the society in which we live. We must continually try to satisfy our needs and yet conform to the demands of our society. We have continually to adapt to other people's needs.

EMOTIONS AND NEEDS

An emotion is a subjective feeling combined with certain bodily changes. Supposing, for instance, you feel afraid, perhaps just before taking an important examination. Your mouth dries up, your heart races, you feel shivery and sweaty and you may keep going to the lavatory. Or you feel angry when someone is rude to you unnecessarily, and again your heart beats faster and your face flushes and your muscles tense. Fear and anger in these circumstances are the appropriate emotions aroused in most people.

Emotions are sparked off by situations which call for the satisfaction of some need. They provide the motivating force behind the actions taken. In an uncomplicated situation fear results in your running away and escaping; anger causes you to attack your opponent with all your strength. But in our society situations are rarely as simple as this. It may be appropriate to run away from an angry lion or to attack an insect that is annoying you. But it is obviously inadvisable to run away before an examination or to attack your boss when he provokes your anger. Most of us have learnt to inhibit and control our behaviour, although we still feel primitive emotions. However, a few unfortunate people seem unable to control themselves and are easily overwhelmed by their emotional impulses. They run away from the examination room or beat up the boss. Inevitably they find themselves in difficulties and do not easily adjust or conform to society.

Once an emotional need has been satisfied, the feeling of discomfort dies away. But adult emotions are often complicated and more than one emotion may be involved at any one time. Conflicting needs can result in tension and discontent.

All needs arouse emotional feelings. But often two or more needs are present at the same time and may conflict with one another. Why, for instance, do most candidates not run from the examination room when their insides 'turn to jelly'? They may be ambitious, and in order to succeed they must pass the examination. They may be conscious of the shame and 'loss of face' that would result from running away. No one likes to be called a coward, to lose the esteem of his companions. For most people the emotion of fear felt before an examination is not strong enough to overcome emotions linked to other needs.

Our sense of identity, the strength of which influences self-confidence and inner security, our values and many of our needs, particularly those concerning relationships with other people, are all acquired in early childhood. How strong these needs are, and the emotional distress that develops when satisfaction is denied them depends partly on the patterns learnt during childhood.

Behaviour can, in fact, be represented diagrammatically by a parallelogram of forces. If an emotion is strong enough it will dominate behaviour until it is satisfied. Take an extreme example, such as the need to breathe, and think what happens when you partially suffocate. You become increasingly afraid, tension builds up and you struggle wildly for breath. If suffocation continues you become panic-stricken and lose all self-control. The bodily accompaniments of fear may last for several minutes after normal breathing has been restored.

The need to breathe is vital for life and cannot be delayed for long. This is why such powerful emotions appear so rapidly and take precedence over any other need at that time. But in a less extreme way emotions are continually determining the way we behave. A heavy smoker who is prevented from smoking for several hours becomes restless, unable to concentrate on his work and is continually searching for an excuse to go out for a cigarette. Many adolescents are dominated by their need for sexual and aggressive outlets, to free themselves from family restrictions. When these needs are frustrated, as they usually are to some degree, the resulting tensions may lead to antisocial behaviour, promiscuity, or the adolescent becoming a 'dropout'. Some men and women, through promiscuity and other ways, are constantly trying to reassure themselves that they are lovable. When such needs are combined with great ability, their lives may be spent in acquiring vast wealth and property, an end in itself rather than a means to other ends.

Emotions also influence what we perceive. A hungry man notices food which he will overlook at other times. Unsatisfied sexual needs can lead to greater awareness of admiring glances or of an attractive pair of legs. Fear can make you more attentive, but it may also bring about a distortion of perception, such as an illusion. Visualize yourself alone at dusk in a house reputed to be haunted. In your frightened state you may easily imagine that a piece of furniture in the shadows is a ghostly figure or that creaks in the hall are footsteps coming towards you.

At one time emotions were thought to be simply the result of becoming aware of internal bodily changes. According to this theory, if you felt afraid it was because of your dry mouth, rapid pulse and other accompaniments of fear; if you felt sad it was because you wept; if you felt hungry it was because your stomach was contracting. This was the *theory of James and Lange*. Although bodily sensations may certainly modify emotional feelings, it seems unlikely that they are responsible for arousing them. There is a good deal of evidence which suggests that emotional feelings arise as a result of activity in the brain itself. Most of the work providing this evidence has been with rats, each with an electrode implanted in a certain area of its brain. Through this a minute stimulating electric current can be given by the rat to itself. Stimulation of certain areas of the brain strongly reinforces behaviour and becomes compulsive; stimulation of other areas has the opposite effect. Human beings, when certain areas of their temporal lobes are stimulated during open brain surgery, have reported intense feelings of pleasure.

Unsatisfied needs lead to emotional feelings and reactions. It is understandable to feel afraid when charging the enemy, or climbing a difficult rock face, or meeting a dangerous animal at large. It is understandable to feel grief at the death of a beloved relative or joy when a much wanted ambition is satisfied. All these emotions are common to most of us in such circumstances.

Other emotions are less easily understood. For instance, a mouse or a spider can hardly be regarded as a real danger, yet in some people they provoke tremendous fear. But mice and spiders can usually be avoided by city dwellers so that even when they arouse strong and uncontrollable emotions they are rarely likely to interfere with everyday life.

But sometimes fear of this type may interfere with everyday life. Suppose, for instance, the fear is for open spaces or for enclosed spaces. Both are common. A fear of open spaces may simply mean that a person avoids going into the country, which probably no one will notice. But if it becomes so extreme that there is fear even of crossing the road, then it is likely to become obvious and seriously to interfere with everyday life. Similarly a fear of enclosed spaces may mean that someone chooses to walk up the stairs instead of using the lift, and this may be regarded as no more than a mild eccentricity. But the fear may be disabling if it leads to an inability to be in a room with the door shut or even in any small room at all.

Fear of some object or situation, for which there is no reasonable cause, is known as a *phobia*. In some cases this can become widespread and crippling, and develop into a *phobic anxiety state*. Sometimes there is no specific phobia, but merely an all-pervading sense of anxiety which seems irrational and ridiculous, yet cannot be shaken off. Such anxiety often stems from a threatened loss of something important in that person's life. Depression follows the actual loss. Such a threat or loss may be real or 'neurotic', meaning that it stems more from inner fantasies than from real outside circumstances. Depression or unhappiness, of course, is felt by everyone at some time or another, following bereavement say, or a serious disappointment. But sometimes depression may be excessive or unaccountably prolonged. It is abnormalities of the emotions like these that constitute psychiatric disorder.

THOUGHT

Thought refers to any conscious mental activity. It can be controlled and directed purposefully as in *reasoning*, or it may be allowed to take its own course as in *fantasy* thinking. McKellar calls these two types of thinking R-thinking, which is logical and reality adjusted, and A-thinking, which is non-rational and is not subject to checking against external events. A-thinking is most clearly seen in dreams, fantasy and some forms of psychotic thinking. For most of us a large part of our daily thought is composed of fantasy.

Imagery may be *visual, auditory, kinaesthetic;* in fact, it may involve any of the senses. People vary in the type they most use. One person may be able to recall clearly a picture of what he was doing yesterday. Another may have only a hazy visual image but be able to 'hear' distinctly what was said at tea-time last week. Yet another may picture a game of tennis or football in terms of body movements and sensations. A peculiarly vivid form of visual imagery occurs in children, almost like photography. This is eidetic imagery and tends to disappear in adult life. Oscar Wilde probably possessed eidetic imagery and as a result was able to mystify people at parties by glancing at a book and then reproducing any part requested.

Much of our thinking occurs in the form of words. For this most of us use auditory rather than visual imagery, but thought can occur without the use of any form of imagery. *Abstract thinking*, for instance on a philosophical problem connected with beauty or goodness, is particularly likely to occur without imagery. The thinker is then simply *aware* of the train of thought.

Reasoning is mainly concerned with solving problems. It involves not only thought but memory and learning. Thought starts when the problem is recognized and continues until it is abandoned or solved. Reasoning is characterized by controlled purposeful thinking which excludes irrelevant thoughts and distractions. The need to solve the problem provides the drive motivating the train of thought. When interest flags concentration and persistence diminish. However, it is important to recognize that in practice rational thought and fantasy thinking are rarely clearly separated. The answer to a problem which has hitherto seemed insoluble may suddenly come during a period of relaxation when thoughts are allowed to wander. Most creative artists and scientists have gained sudden insight into their work on waking from a night's sleep. Fantasy thinking is intimately bound up with creativity.

Rational thought, concentration and memory are usually disturbed by the presence of strong emotional factors, particularly tension. Serious psychiatric disorder also distorts rational thinking.

FANTASY OR AUTISTIC THOUGHT. Fantasy thinking, unlike reasoning, occurs without conscious control or direction. It may well be that fantasy thinking represents some base line of activity of the brain, just as during sleep some degree of dreaming always seems to be occurring, whatever the depth of sleep. All of us indulge in fantasy thinking—for instance, day-dreaming—at some time during the day. During such fantasy thinking you are largely cut off from the outside world and from reality. Freud looked upon daydreams and dreaming as 'wish fulfilments' unconsciously directed. Fantasy thoughts certainly provide an outlet for bottled-up aggression and frustrations. Indeed, fantasy is a tremendous safety valve, by means of which we can experience socially forbidden or impossible activities with ease and safety. Fantasy thinking will also give satisfaction to more prosaic needs. On a cold, wet winter day you can dream of the Mediterranean. A hungry man enjoys thinking of food, the thirsty one of sparkling waters, the sexually frustrated of sex. The person who feels a failure in his work dreams of success and acclaim. There is no harm in this unless fantasy takes the place of reality and interferes with adaptation, as it may do in some forms of psychopathy and mental illness.

Fantasy develops in a child along with memory. During the first three or four years fantasy is probably inseparable from the child's play. But from then on, play becomes gradually more 'socialized' and the two slowly begin to diverge. Fantasy thinking reaches its peak in puberty and is particularly likely to have a sexual colouring, or to be concerned with ambitions. Although fantasy does not generally produce action, adolescent fantasy thinking may provide additional incentives for working and passing exams, and in increasing social activities and confidence.

Sexual fantasies, those connected with masturbation and sexual intercourse, are of particular interest. They involve sadomasochistic themes, and they inversely reflect outward personality traits. They are particularly important, not only in understanding sexual deviations, but also in understanding normal sexual relationships and the difficulties that may arise within marriage. (See p. 59.)

Fantasy thinking and dreaming are closely related, and one may fade into the other on going to sleep or on waking. Fantasy thinking is increased by anxiety or by any condition which interferes with rational thought. Drugs such as marijuana and alcohol, amphetamines and some of the psychotropic drugs (although this will also depend upon the type of personality of the patient) can all enhance fantasy thinking.

MEMORY

What is memory? What happens when you try to memorize a poem, or the causes of heart failure, or the ways of bandaging a hand? Why is it so much more difficult to memorize a meaningless jumble of words or numbers than a poem or something which makes sense?

Not only is memory made up of several different mental functions, but there is a difference between long- and short-term memory. Much of what we see or hear needs to be remembered only for a short time, and can then be forgotten. For instance, a telephonist needs to remember a number only for a minute or so; if she tried to memorize numbers for longer, she would soon be in a muddle. Short-term memory is said to involve an 'activity trace', a kind of mirror image of events, which rapidly decays.

Anything committed to memory must first be learnt. The information is then *stored or retained* in the brain, although how this is done is not known. We suppose that some physical change must accompany the imprinting of information on the brain. We call this supposed change a *memory* or *structural* trace. When we wish to remember something, the relevant memory is activated and brought into consciousness. This is known as *recall*. Provided the correct memory trace has been recalled, its appearance in consciousness is accompanied by a sense of recognition. If it is wrong, it is rejected.

Sometimes information may be forgotten, either temporarily or permanently. We have all had the experience of meeting an old friend and being unable to recall his name. Perhaps you have experienced stagefright and forgotten completely the lines you knew by heart so perfectly only a few minutes earlier. The information is still there, since it will certainly be remembered later. In this case anxiety has interfered with recall.

Anxious and agitated patients often experience similar difficulties in recalling recently acquired information. Drugs also interfere with recall, particularly amphetamines and the monoamine oxidase inhibitor group of antidepressants.

The psychologist Thorndike believed that forgetting occurred as a result of *trace decay*, of memories fading through disuse. But this now seems unlikely to be true. Recent evidence, both clinical and experimental, suggests that forgotten memories have become inaccessible rather than decayed. New memories often interfere with old ones. Loss of memory may be due more to '*retroactive inhibition*' than to time itself. Retroactive inhibition is the interference with a memory trace in the brain that occurs as a result of the later learning of similar information. For example, you may remember a shopping list perfectly all day, but after you have learnt the next day's shopping list, you may be unable to remember the first.

Retroactive inhibition ceases during sleep. For this reason the best time to learn something that you really want to remember is just before you go to bed, as there will then be plenty of time for the information to fix itself firmly in the memory, without interference.

DEVELOPMENT OF MEMORY. Memory develops slowly and by stages. A baby of a month or two will smile at his mother, but this is a reflex response to her face, and he will smile just as well if he is shown a paper mask. At this age the child is still unable to *recognize* his mother.

The ability to recognize develops before the ability to *recall*. By the time he is six months old the baby is able to recognize his mother and other people around him, his own hands and feet and his toys in the cot. But he is still unable to recall his mother and familiar beings and objects in their absence. He still lives entirely in the present. Recall becomes possible at about the end of a child's first year of life. He can now remember where he puts his toys, even though they are not visible. He can also visualize his mother when she is not present. At first the process of recall is unstable, and he can only think back a few minutes. But this interval grows progressively longer, and by the age of four he can recall events that occurred months or as long as a year ago. Past learning can now be recalled for solving new problems and developing conceptual thought.

Memory is not a static process by means of which information is photographed, stored and reproduced unchanged some time later. Memory is an active process, and memories are continually being inhibited, forgotten, modified and distorted. Just as perceptual processes tend to fill in gaps and to reduce unfamiliar perceptions to more familiar and conventional ones, so also memory is biased towards what is familiar. We spoke of the recall of a trace memory, but of course in practice recall is never as simple as this. Trace memories are continually modified by related experiences and emotional attitudes. Recollections are always liable to this type of distortion, and the longer the time between the event and the recall, the greater is the distortion. Unpleasant memories are liable to be *repressed*, particularly those liable to cause anxiety. The conscious reliving of some

repressed incident, by hypnosis or giving the patient intravenous metho-hexitone sodium or sodium amytal, is sometimes used in the treatment of psychological disorders. Such a method of treatment is known as *abreaction*.
THE PHYSICAL BASIS OF MEMORY. We still know very little about the physical basis of memory. Hebb's two-stage theory of memory postulates that incoming stimulation sets up reverberatory activity in and between the receptor and effector cells involved. With repeated stimulation and reverberation, structural changes occur, setting up a memory or structural trace. Electric shocks might be expected to interfere with this process, and certainly can be shown to do so in the case of rats. Electro-convulsive therapy (E.C.T.) sometimes has a disruptive effect on recent memory, particularly when given bilaterally. (See p. 187.)

Visual hallucinations may occur during epileptic disturbances arising from the occipitoparietal area of the cerebral cortex. Vivid memories can also be produced by electrical stimulation of certain parts of the temporal lobe of the brain. From a structural point of view the limbic lobe (see p. 73) seems to be intimately involved with memory. In the *Korsakov Syndrome*, a complication of alcoholism, the patient cannot form new memories or recall recent events. In this condition lesions are found in the *mammillary bodies* and the medial thalamus. The *hippocampus* is linked to the *mammillary bodies* by the fornix. Apart from damage to the *mammillary bodies*, bilateral removal or damage to the *hippocampus*, or surgical section of the fornix, will produce similar disturbances of memory. Temporal lobectomy can be followed by profound amnesia going back several years.

Chemical changes in the brain may also be related to memory. Ribonu-cleic acid (RNA) has been extracted from the brains of animals trained in certain tasks and injected into untrained animals. It has been claimed that 'memories' have been transferred by this means from trained to untrained animals. This work is still very much in its infancy and experi-mental results are not easy to interpret.

Patients with *temporal lobe epilepsy* may experience *déjà vu*, a curious sense of familiarity that they have 'been here before' or lived through the same experience at some earlier stage of existence. This sense of familiarity is never complete and delusions rarely arise. The feeling is experienced by normal people, particularly when fatigued or worried. It can result from the use of certain drugs, particularly marijuana and hallucinogenic drugs, occasionally from excessive use of alcohol. In acute anxiety states it may be associated with depersonalization. It is a not uncommon symptom in acute psychotic states.

For memory tests, see p. 94.

LEARNING

We start to learn as soon as we are born, if not before. How we behave as adults is largely determined by what we learn in our early years. In more ways than one the child is father to the man.

The baby learns that his mother will satisfy his needs. He learns to be clean, and to behave in ways that are acceptable to others. He learns to crawl and walk, to ride a bicycle, to solve arithmetical problems, to recognize danger, and so on. All learning is concerned with adapting to new situations and problems. Compared with some other animals the human child is born with few instinctive forms of behaviour. His nervous system is like plasticine, waiting to be moulded by environmental influences.

There is still a good deal of disagreement about how learning actually occurs. Much of our information comes from experiments with animals, particularly rats, and it is not always easy to know how much of it applies to humans.

IMPRINTING. Very rapid learning in animals occurs at certain times during development. The nervous system needs to have developed and to be ready to respond to the stimulus encountered. The learning process is rapid, tenacious and long lasting. This form of learning was studied by Konrad Lorenz in birds, and in its original sense imprinting referred to the attachment which newly hatched birds develop to moving objects, living or inanimate, in their immediate vicinity. Lorenz's early work was with mallard ducklings and grey-legged goslings. They quickly learned to follow the first moving object they encountered (usually of course the mother duck or goose) and thereafter would only follow the imprinted 'object'. Lorenz showed that the adult sexual behaviour of these birds was also influenced by this early imprinting. There is however controversy as to whether such sexual imprinting arises from the initial imprinting phenomenon or whether it develops separately.

It seems possible that imprinting plays a part in human development and behaviour, both sexual and non-sexual.

CLASSICAL CONDITIONING. Relatively simple learning is based on the principle of the conditioned reflex. The Russian physiologist Pavlov was the first to make a detailed study of conditioned reflexes, although it had long been known that two events occurring together in time tend to become linked in the mind. Pavlov studied unconditioned reflexes in dogs, particularly the reflex that causes saliva to drip from the lips when meat is placed in the dog's mouth. He found that when another stimulus, a light or a bell, was given with the meat several times running, the dog would sooner or later produce saliva on this stimulus alone and without the meat. The light or bell had thus become a *conditioned stimulus*, and the salivation that followed when it was given was known as a *conditioned reflex*. The conditioned stimulus had to be reinforced from time to time by combining it with food, otherwise the conditioned reflex tended to fade.

Pavlov put forward a theory of two complementary processes in the nervous system. (1) A process of excitation spreads through the nervous system as conditioned reflexes form. (2) A process of inhibition develops when stimuli are not reinforced, so that eventually no response occurs to them. Pavlov's theory has been utilized and elaborated upon by William

Sargant in *Battle for the Mind,* which purports to explain certain types of behaviour.

Pavlov's work was taken up and applied in an extreme way to human learning by Watson, an American psychologist. He virtually rejected the idea of anything being inherited through the central nervous system. He declared that an infant is born with a few simple reflexes only, and that these reflex responses become linked to new stimuli by conditioning, and grow steadily more complex. He believed that by proper conditioning

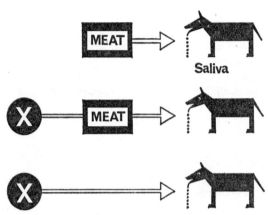

Saliva

FIGURE 1.1

any child could successfully be brought up to be anything you chose, whether this be a doctor, soccer star or dustman.

It now seems most unlikely that all human behaviour and learning can be explained simply on the basis of conditioned reflexes. However, conditioning does give an acceptable explanation of some of it.

Classical conditioning also gives an acceptable explanation of how certain irrational fears and dislikes may develop through emotional responses of the autonomic nervous system becoming associated with objects or situations. Watson carried out a famous experiment on a small boy called Albert. He showed him a white rat, and at the same time frightened him by making a loud noise. He repeated this on several occasions, and eventually the boy became afraid of the rat, and cried whenever he saw it. His fear spread to include all white furry animals, and Albert went out of his way to avoid them. White furry animals had become a conditioned stimulus which caused fear. In everyday language he had learnt to fear and to avoid such animals. Many of us have equally absurd fears connected with mice, insects or birds, which we have probably learned like little Albert.

LEARNING BY TRIAL AND ERROR. This is more usually known as instrumental or *operant conditioning.* Conditioning is built upon operant behaviour, that is on the normal activities of the animal. Instrumental or

13

operant conditioning consists of rewarding and/or punishing some acts and not others, thereby directing the animal's behaviour in a certain direction. This is based on Thorndike's law of effect. Thorndike showed if you shut up a hungry cat in a suitable cage with food placed on the floor outside, the cat stretches and pulls at the bars of the cage until eventually by chance it releases the catch holding the door. Next day the same behaviour may occur, but eventually the cat goes straight to the catch and opens the door. The initial opening of the cage is by chance, but since this action results in satisfying the cat's needs by reducing its hunger, the cat quickly learns to release the catch whenever it is put into the cage. Thorndike's law of effect states that actions which result in satisfaction become stronger, while those which cause no satisfaction are weakened and eventually ignored.

Various methods are available for studying operant conditioning. In the Skinner box the animal learns to obtain food or water by pressing a lever or by some analogous action. In the T-maze the animal has to find the right turning. Operant learning may be based on a reward system or punishment training.

Both classical and operant conditioning need reinforcement. Whereas in classical conditioning the unconditioned stimulus is the reinforcement, in operant conditioning the reinforcing stimulus is associated with and follows some particular response.

Every mother and school child knows the principle of operant conditioning, the rewards of 'good' behaviour, the punishment of 'bad' behaviour. This is the basis of much of the upbringing, training and education of children, of how they learn to behave and acquire simple skills. The reward need not necessarily be a material one. The approval of someone whom the child loves and respects may be just as good as, if not better than material rewards.

LEARNING WITH INSIGHT. The idea that learning can be achieved by trial and error has been much criticized on the grounds that learning is then entirely automatic. This may well be so in lower animals, but in man and the higher apes *understanding* and *insight* are also involved. Kohler showed that chimpanzees were able to solve problems by piling boxes on top of one another or fitting sticks together in an insightful way.

A small child seems to learn at first by trial and error, which is probably a reflection of the child's lack of experience. But before long he adopts a more rational approach to new problems. He no longer acts by trial and error, but picks out helpful facts which may help him to solve the problem by linking it up with what he has already learnt.

Man can learn much more quickly and efficiently than other animals because he has the use of language. By means of words he can think out ways of tackling new problems, selecting only those ways which seem likely to succeed. This, of course, is a sort of mental trial and error, but it is very different from the trial and error behaviour of the cat in the cage.

EXPOSURE LEARNING. Apart from classical and operant conditioning it seems likely that learning also occurs without specific reinforcement, simply from exposure to a particular experience. Thus hungry or thirsty rats rapidly learn to run through a maze when rewarded in the end. A satiated and therefore unmotivated rat does not appear to learn, yet if after being allowed to wander at will through the maze he is then motivated, he then learns very quickly. Some people believe in playing classical music as a background to their children's lives, others try to learn a foreign language by playing a tape just before going to sleep, on the same principle.

A number of factors influence learning:

1. *Motivation.* Without motivation there can be no drive to learn. In order to be motivated there must be a need, and therefore an interest in the subject. There may be several conflicting needs, causing ambivalence and indecisiveness over learning. Anxiety sometimes acts as a spur to learning, but if too great its effect is disruptive.

2. *Punishment.* There is still considerable controversy about the value or otherwise of punishment in learning. In general, punishment is an effective instrument for avoidance training, both with animals and man. Thus a child learns to wash his hands before meals because otherwise he will not be allowed to eat at table. However, if punishment is too severe it provokes such anxiety that learning is inhibited. Thus it only makes matters worse if a frightened child is threatened or punished for wetting his bed. In such a case it is better to reward the child for being dry than punishing him for being wet. But many factors are involved in the efficiency of punishment. Punishment is most effective when it immediately follows the response. And from the point of view of a child, it depends upon how he views the punishment, how consistent, restrictive or permissive his parents and other authority figures are towards him.

3. *Positive reinforcement.* This is rewarding an action which strengthens the likelihood that it will be performed again, according to the *law of effect* (see p. 14).

4. *Exercise and repetition.* This will increase the rate of learning. *Over-learning*, continuing the learning process for longer than is necessary, fixes what has been learnt more securely in the brain.

PERCEPTION

Perception is a process by which we become aware of what is happening around us and in our own bodies. But it is more than just receiving stimuli through our special sense organs: eyes, ears, skin and so on. It is more than just recording stimuli. Perception is an active process of the brain which selects and organizes stimuli. The selection and organization are performed according to inherent properties of the brain and past learning and experience. They are thus also influenced by interest, needs and emotions. In a way you can compare this internal perceptual process with what happens when a lump of clay is modelled. The final result depends upon the structure of the clay and the skill of the modeller, together with his interest and feelings at the time. The lump of clay will be transformed according to all these things. So also do perceptual processes deal with stimuli that reach the brain and transform them into recognizable objects and scenes. These objects and scenes are then *projected* out of the brain and back into the environment.

Each growing individual has to learn the *meaning* of *stimuli* or *signs*. A child gradually learns to recognize objects, distance, time and so on by experience. He does this by exploring his environment constantly, by handling and reaching for objects. All the time he is combining and comparing what he sees with what he feels and hears. He perceives adults and learns that a smile means approval or happiness, and a frown disapproval. He observes closely how people behave in different circumstances and learns to perceive their attitudes and purpose from their expressions and behaviour. As he learns to understand words his development is helped by language.

William James, a famous psychologist of the last century, thought that a new-born child saw the world as 'blooming, buzzing confusion'. This is probably wrong for it is unlikely that the new-born child is aware of anything except himself, and he is probably incapable of distinguishing himself from things outside himself. For the new-born infant existence probably consists largely of his needs, and whether or not these needs are satisfied. However, the world may well appear to be all confusion to a man, blind from birth, whose vision is suddenly restored by an operation. Imagine you know him well and are by his bedside when the bandages are removed from his eyes for the first time. Do you think he will smile and say, 'You look just as I expected'? On the contrary, although he knows who and where you are from your voice, he will see you only as a blur, without expression, colour or distinguishing features. The receptors in his retina are responding to you, but the impulses travelling from them to his brain are as yet meaningless. Only after a time, with experience and learning, will he come to recognize your features and be able to distinguish you from someone else. Even after learning to recognize you in the hospital ward he may fail to recognize you at first in unfamiliar surroundings. For such a man visual learning is very slow compared with that of a child.

It is probable that, as with other functions, there is a *critical period of development* during which perceptual learning is most effective. If, for one reason or another, perception is interfered with during this critical period, subsequent learning is much slower and less effective. We can compare this with what happens in chickens. It is obviously important that chicks should be able to peck efficiently. Experiments suggest that there is a critical period coinciding with the first fourteen days after hatching during which the chick must have pecking experience if he is to develop his powers of pecking adequately. If he is prevented from pecking during the first fourteen days of his life the bird is permanently retarded in pecking compared with its fellow chicks.

But not all perception is due to learning. The internal processes involved in perception depend also on inherent properties of the brain. Much of our knowledge of these inherent properties comes from the work of *Gestalt* (meaning form or pattern) psychologists working in the early half of this century. These workers saw that the perceptual field was organized in such a way that certain unitary parts stood out as wholes; and these segregated themselves from the rest of the field. Thus three dots on a sheet of paper forms a triangle.

If more dots are added the triangle is eventually lost. Such a segregated whole is called a *Gestalt*, from which the *Gestalt theory* is derived. The

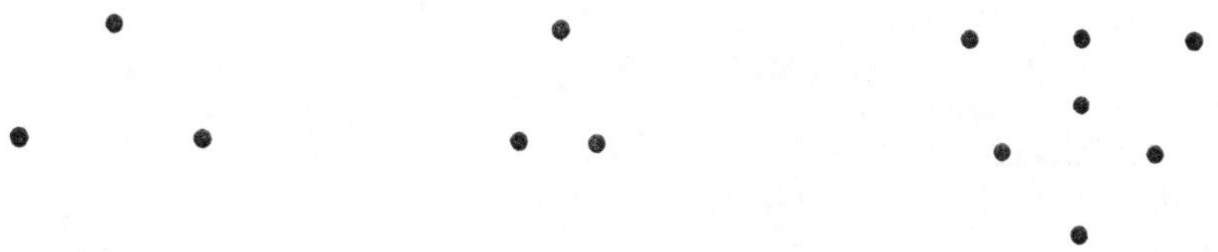

FIGURE 1.2

distinguishing characteristic of a *Gestalt* is that the segregated whole (in this case the triangle) is more than simply the sum of its parts. As you can see (Fig. 1.2), the shape varies although the parts remain the same.

The way dots become organized into *Gestalten* is determined by their closeness to one another, by their similarity in shape and size, and by their continuity of direction. No matter what it is perceiving, the brain tends as far as possible to perceive the most simple and stable geometrical shapes in preference to unstable complicated shapes.

When a child is faced with an unfamiliar jumble of stimuli, he first tends to pick out some bright spot or moving object that stands out from its background. A figure stands out naturally against a shapeless background; for instance, a black triangle drawn on a white piece of paper is sharply outlined. But if the figure is not too different from its background, its contour may be indistinct and it will then be *unstable* and will keep disappearing into the background. This, of course, is the principle upon which camouflage is based and it also accounts for ghostly appearances at dusk.

Another characteristic of the brain is *perceptual constancy*. The size, shape, brightness and colour of anything remains constant. When you see a man at a distance of a hundred yards the image he makes on your retina must be smaller than the image of a man only ten yards away; yet you will perceive them both as of similar size (see Fig. 1.3). Because of its previous experience in these matters your brain automatically adjusts its interpretation of the actual image that is received according to the estimated distance.

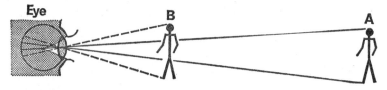

FIGURE 1.3

Similarly you will perceive a coin as round whether you look at it face to face or end on. Your experience tells you that it is round and so you perceive it as such. This perceptual constancy produces a basically stable world within which you can appreciate perceptual changes. Without such constancy the external world would seem to be unbearably chaotic.

We mentioned earlier that subjective factors influence perception. For instance, you easily pick out a familiar figure in a crowd, particularly if you expect to see him. There is a tendency to overlook mistakes in familiar material. You may for instance not see glaring errors in your own writing. People fill in details according to what they expect to find. This often happens in a Court of Law. A witness may, unwittingly and in all honesty, fill in gaps in his account of what happened, and the brain may alter the story itself in various ways to make it conform to what is familiar and expected. For this reason two witnesses may, and often do, give honest but completely different accounts of an accident.

Emotional attitudes and habits also have considerable influence. If you are afraid or suspicious you are liable to see other people as unfriendly, and to misinterpret innocent remarks and gestures as though they were directed against you. In extreme cases, usually associated with psychiatric illness, a man may misinterpret remarks and gestures so grossly that he may even assault total strangers violently, believing them to be hostile to him.

Stereotypes are groups of fixed, over-simplified and generalized conceptions that many individuals have about other people, such as the latin races, negroes, the working-class, civil servants, nurses. When these conceptions are unfavourable they are linked with *prejudice*. Many people, not least among the medical and nursing professions, have a stereotyped idea of mental illness. They see the mentally ill as dangerous, unable to control their feelings and morally blameworthy.

Prejudice influences how one person perceives another, and how he behaves towards him. A Nazi who knew a man was a Jew might perceive him to be a loathsome villain and exterminate him without mercy. Yet such a man could be kind and considerate to non-Jews. Similar prejudices exist today towards men of different colour and race. Most of us have minor prejudices about the way people speak or eat, certain forms of dress or hair-style, foods and so on, which affect our attitudes and feelings. Many of our prejudices are based not so much on ignorance as upon fear and our own sense of insecurity. The homosexual patient may be disliked because of the fear he arouses.

Emotions can influence perception in negative as well as in positive ways. Unpleasant incidents are overlooked or conveniently forgotten. If you happen to meet someone you dislike you may fail to recognize him. Or you may misread the date of a dreaded interview and arrive a day late for it.

There is continual rejection and selection of stimuli by the brain. Sometimes perception may be so distorted that an *illusion* is produced. This occurs either because the stimuli are misleading or ambiguous, or because the internal organization of the brain has broken down. *Illusions* are *errors of perception* which cause stimuli to be wrongly interpreted. We mentioned above how extreme fear or anger, especially when there is lack of perceptual clarity, may do this. Some old people at night, and delirious patients, are particularly liable to suffer from illusions; a piece of fluff on the bed may become a terrifying animal, a nurse becomes a threatening intruder. Illusions and hallucinations are common in the early stages of bereavement: the dead person is heard coming into the house or even speaking, and may perhaps be glimpsed in the hall or the bedroom at twilight. It is important to recognize that illusions are not necessarily morbid, and that any of us can experience illusions if conditions are appropriate.

Hallucinations are even more abnormal for these are perceptions that arise without any stimuli at all, and so they can only be perceived by the patient and cannot be shared with others. Often *hallucinations* only occur or are most troublesome at night when external stimuli are least. It seems as though the brain has a need for stimulation in order to relate itself adequately to its environment. In *sensory deprivation experiments* volunteers have been cut off, as far as possible, from all sensory stimuli. As a result, normal people have developed *illusions* and *hallucinations*. Oldish patients operated upon for cataract, who have their eyes bandaged for several days post-operatively, not infrequently hallucinate. Rather similar experiences have been described by arctic explorers, long-distance drivers and shipwreck survivors at sea. In these people *hallucinations* and *illusions* sometimes seem to occur as a result of monotony and a lack of fresh stimulation. Hallucinations may involve any of the senses. Many normal people experience hallucinations as they are falling asleep or waking; these are known as hypnogogic and hypnopompic hallucinations respectively. Auditory hallucinations are more common than visual, and usually take the form of the subject's name being called. Volunteers deprived of sleep may develop a *hypnogogic psychosis*, with auditory and visual hallucinations. Auditory hallucinations, in a setting of clear consciousness, are characteristic of schizophrenia. Patients with severe psychotic depression sometimes report hearing disjointed words or phrases. Visual hallucinations are common in delirium and states of intoxication, and are not uncommon in hysteria. Temporal lobe lesions can cause visual hallucinations and hallucinations of smell and taste.

Reality. We have explained how perception involves receiving and reorganizing stimuli and projecting them back into the environment. We have also mentioned that errors of perception may arise and a man may hear voices and see forms which no one else can hear or see.

How do we know that what we perceive has physical reality? Most of us take this for granted. What we perceive is familiar and fits into our framework of *reality*. Moreover, as far as we can see, it is accepted and shared by other people. But if we see a devil sitting at the foot of the bed or hear threatening voices coming from the radiator, we are puzzled and frightened. These perceptions are *unreal*, particularly as no one else can see or hear them. But if we go on having these perceptions for some time we may come to accept them as real. When this happens, as in *schizophrenia*, *sense of reality* is lost and adaptation to the environment becomes disturbed, particularly social relationships.

However, it is important to realize that there is no absolute reality. We all have our own personal fantasy world which exists and interacts with what is going on in the outside world. When we are extremely tense, confused, intoxicated, mentally ill, inner fantasies may become for a time more real than what is happening in the outside world.

DEVELOPMENT OF PERCEPTION OF SELF. Perception develops along with thinking and memory. At first there is little distinction between self and the external world. Even before birth tactile sensations are constantly travelling from different parts of the body to the brain. After birth, as a child becomes more mobile, he gradually increases his knowledge of his body from tactile sensations. He explores his body with his hands and his self-awareness increases. Vision, hearing, pain, temperature and smell play their part. He develops an awareness of himself and his *body image*. As he grows and increases his activities, his mental picture of himself is continually modified. Emotional attitudes and values become attached to this image of his body and its various parts. The attitude of his parents, his relationship with them, and his early childhood experiences inevitably influence to some extent the way he regards himself. Strength and muscular development, beauty, intellectual prowess, or chastity may be praised or devalued according to family values. A man may put tremendous significance on the physical development of his body and spend all his spare time playing games and doing gymnastics. For such a man to be physically disabled by illness or injury, however minor the disability, may be catastrophic and result in severe psychiatric disturbance.

Adults who lose a limb commonly experience the sensation that it is still present. This imaginary limb is known as a *phantom limb*. It is interesting that children born without limbs, or who lose a limb before the age of five, do not develop phantom limbs. Presumably the *body image* is not yet properly formed.

Organic factors may form the basis of some symptoms which may be labelled psychiatric. Thus the child may be damaged in utero or suffer some minor injury at birth, insufficient to cause cerebral palsy but sufficient to cause sensory deficiencies and interfere with his development and co-ordination. As a result he may be late in learning to read or write, excessively clumsy, unable to ride a bike and so on. The body-image concept normally arises in the second half of the first year and only when this is established can the child respond as a whole appropriately to afferent stimuli. If the body image concept is deficient the child will find it difficult to wash, walk, feed, dress and carry out the most basic functions. A vicious circle may clearly spring up as a result of this and the child may be looked upon as psychiatrically disturbed and his disabilities attributed to this rather than vice versa.

Both constitutional factors and learning are involved in the development of perception. For instance, infants begin to follow the movements of their hands with their eyes from about twelve weeks. This is so even in children blind from birth. But if there is no feedback, the co-ordination of eyes and hands gradually ceases. The child has to compensate through other senses, such as hearing, touch, taste, which may become more developed than normal.

Congenitally deaf children will have difficulty with speech. They begin to babble like other children from about three months old, but because they cannot hear themselves or others, learning cannot naturally take over from the babbling stage.

Children have enormous potential for adapting. Thalidomide children, born without limbs, are able to adapt perceptually so well that they are just as competent as normal children on intelligence testing at the age of two. Children with sensory or physical defects need above all to feel secure in order to develop and compensate to the full. Parents of such children may be guilty and ashamed, ignorant of how to help their child. They will often need prolonged support. The child must not be over-protected, for he needs new experiences in order to develop. And to learn he needs the incentive of praise and encouragement from those he loves and respects.

SEXUAL IDENTITY. (GENDER IDENTITY).   Most of us are labelled boy or girl correctly at birth, the form of our external genitalia reflecting the appropriate internal reproductive system, hormones, and chromosomes. Rarely a mistake is made, and the child whose chromosomes and hormones are male is brought up as a female, or vice versa. Usually, but not invariably, if and when a mistake is discovered the child chooses to retain the sexual role to which he has become accustomed.

From a *psychosexual* point of view, are we born male or female, or are we 'neutral' at birth, everything depending upon upbringing? Childhood experiences are certainly major factors in shaping sexual identity. But there is now evidence for believing that intrauterine influences, especially the effect of foetal androgens on developing hypothalamic centres, may be important, so that at birth the child is predisposed to develop as male or female. Psychological differences undoubtedly exist between the two sexes at birth, but many of the differences which later develop are largely due to variations in the upbringing of boys and girls.

It is important to distinguish between a person's sexual identity, his choice of sexual object, and his sexual drive. A male may have no doubts about his maleness for instance, but is only sexually attracted to another male. This is discussed in more detail in Sexual Deviations.

2

INTELLIGENCE

Intelligence has different meanings for different people. To an educator it probably means the *ability to learn*; to a biologist it may be the *capacity to adapt*; while psychologists use the word intelligence to mean the *ability to reason* and to think rationally and purposefully. It is the capacity to use experience and knowledge that constitutes intelligent behaviour and enables man to solve problems and to adapt to changing situations. You can, for instance, give a man a perfect set of tools; but unless he has the necessary intelligence, he will never acquire the skill that is necessary to use those tools.

Intelligent behaviour is always rational. It differs greatly from instinctive or impulsive behaviour which may seem pointless and harmful. Consider the behaviour of a man who is trying to cross a river. First, he looks for a bridge or a boat; in the absence of these he tries to find a shallow crossing; failing this he starts to build himself a raft, and so on. This behaviour is rational and understandable. But compare this to the behaviour of a wealthy woman who had a quarrel with her husband, went out to a shop, stole a cheap trinket, and was caught and sent to prison. Such impulsive behaviour is purposeless and not understandable at first sight. What is more, it is unadaptable, for it may be repeated time after time, showing that no lesson has been learnt from the experience.

But it is usually impossible entirely to distinguish intelligent from impulsive behaviour. Most human action is, in fact, a mixture of both. Unconscious impulses may provide the drive for apparently intelligent behaviour, and much of our everyday behaviour is based upon habit, prejudices, and emotional likes and dislikes of which we are often hardly aware.

Intelligence often develops unevenly in the growing child and reaches its maximum usually at about the age of fifteen or sixteen, though perhaps a few years later in some people. It is important to realize that although intelligence is maximum, experience and knowledge are not. Moreover, an adolescent often has limited control over his impulses. Thus, to an adult, adolescent behaviour often seems to be irrational.

As age advances intelligence declines, and this decline is probably slower in people who use their minds. Old people find it harder to learn, and they cannot adapt so readily to change as young people.

In the past fifty years many tests have been developed in an attempt to provide an objective measurement of intelligence. Alfred Binet worked with Paris school children and was the originator of these tests. He decided that no single test could measure intelligence and he therefore designed a variety of different tests, using the obvious fact that children become more 'clever' with age. He found that the *average* child at each age could do certain things. For instance, a three-year-old could string at least four beads in two minutes; a six-year-old could count thirteen coins, copy a diamond shape, and see what is missing in pictures of incomplete faces; a nine-year-old could describe how wood and coal are alike and how they differ.

Binet tried out his tests on many children and modified them until he eventually knew which could be done by the majority of children in each age-group. The modern *Binet–Simon scale* contains 55 tests. This is made up of five items for each year from 3–10 inclusive, 12, 15, and an adult group. The age-group for which the child passes *all* tests is known as the *basal age*; to this is added the number of tests that the child can pass for higher ages. The total gives the *mental age*. For instance, let us consider the performance of a 6-year-old child.

4-year tests — 5 *out of 5 tests passed* = basal age
5-year test — 3 out of 5 tests passed
6-year test — 2 out of 5 tests passed
7-year test — 0 out of 5 tests passed
Mental Age = basal age $(4) + (\frac{3}{5} + \frac{2}{5})$ = 5 years

This is then expressed as the *intelligence quotient* (I.Q.). This is the ratio of

$$\frac{\text{mental age}}{\text{chronological age}} \times 100$$

In this case the I.Q. is $\frac{5}{6} \times 100 = 83$

The *average* child of six has an I.Q. of $\frac{6}{6} \times 100 = 100$. This child is therefore well below the *average intelligence* of six-year-olds. In practice, the term 'average' includes everyone with an I.Q. of between 90 and 110.

Numerous tests of intelligence have been designed since Binet's work was published. Tests in common use today are the Stanford–Binet scale for children between 2 and 18, and the Wechsler intelligence scale for children (W.I.S.C.). For testing of adults the Wechsler Bellevue scale is preferable, the I.Q. being calculated by comparing the actual score with the expected average score of adults of the same age.

I.Q. tests are reasonably reliable in that they give a similar result on retesting. However, variations of up to 15–20 points can occur over a five-year period, particularly with a bright child. The I.Q. is mainly a measure of a child's present status, in relation to children of similar age, and not necessarily a reliable pointer to his future abilities. The growth of intelligence is not a smooth upward curve but consists of spurts and plateaux which may continue into late adolescence. I.Q. tests measure only what they set out to measure. Nonetheless the I.Q. correlates positively with actual intellectual activity and scholastic ability, and is a useful practical measure of a person's intelligence.

The Stanford–Binet and the W.I.S.C. scales are composed of groups of verbal and non-verbal, or performance tests. Verbal tests include general knowledge, comprehension, arithmetical problems, the ability to recognize similarities and dissimilarities, vocabulary range and digit span. Their solution depends to a large degree on a child's education and upbringing. Performance tests, which include assembling jigsaws, completing missing parts of pictures, paper-and-pencil maze tests, are less dependent on educational and cultural factors for their solution. Most people score roughly the same on verbal and performance tests. A marked discrepancy between verbal and performance test scores may result from lack of education, unrecognized deafness or other perceptual deficiencies, psychosis or brain injury. In such cases the child's uneven abilities are liable to create uncertainty and anxiety, both in him and in his parents, which may result later in psychiatric problems.

A number of other factors, apart from cultural, can affect I.Q. test results. A child may lack motivation to complete the test, extreme anxiety interferes with his understanding and performance of the test. Practice in I.Q. tests adds only about 5 points, but frequent coaching can increase an I.Q. score by as much as 15–20 points.

Group tests are given to several individuals at once and do not require skilled supervision. For this reason among others, they are less reliable than individual tests. Achievement tests are group tests which measure and compare one child with another in terms of school subjects. The I.Q. of children under two can be measured by Ruth Griffith's mental development scale. This assesses the child's locomotor development, learning and speech, hand and eye co-ordination and his personal social adjustment. The tester must be specially trained.

Various theories exist as to what exactly is being measured by intelligence tests. Spearman believed that individual differences in tests were due to the presence of one factor common to all tests, which he labelled G or general intelligence, and others specific to the tests involved.

DISTRIBUTION OF I.Q. IN THE POPULATION

The distribution of I.Q. in a population is, for a large sample, a 'normal' one. That is, if the number of people of similar I.Q. scores is plotted on the scale of intelligence, a symmetrical curve is obtained (slightly skewed to the lower end of intelligence). This suggests that variations in intelligence, like stature and weight, are dependent on many small effects, genetic and/or environmental, opposing or reinforcing one another. Above an

I.Q. of 50 the genetic effects are thought to be due to multifactorial genes scattered throughout the normal population. Below an I.Q. of about 50, single pathological genes, chromosomal defects, infections of and injury to the brain, are more likely to be responsible.

Figure 2.1 shows the distribution of I.Q. throughout the population. I.Q. is sometimes expressed as a percentile. An individual with an I.Q. of 130 is more intelligent than 96 per cent of the population and therefore falls above the 96th percentile. An I.Q. of between 90 and 110 is regarded as 'average'. 55 per cent of the population fall within this range. To go

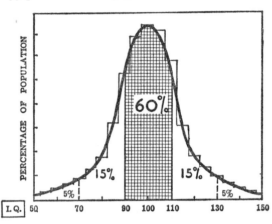

FIGURE 2.1

into the professional classes you need an I.Q. of at least 110. Only 1 per cent have an I.Q. above 140. To go to University it is advisable to have an I.Q. of 120 or above.

Education may be a problem in children of very high intelligence. They easily become bored and ordinary education may not give them enough intellectual stimulation. Yet moving them into a class of older children may be difficult, for their *emotional development* may not be sufficiently great to enable them to adjust to older children. Children with average, or with slightly above average I.Q., who scrape into Grammar Schools, may be pushed too hard by over-ambitious parents. Educational difficulties may also occur in the child of *border-line subnormality* (see p. 171) who is unable to cope in an ordinary school. He may become a behaviour problem until he is transferred to a *school for educationally subnormal children*.

THE INFLUENCE OF HEREDITY AND ENVIRONMENT ON INTELLIGENCE

Differences of intelligence between different people are largely due to *genetic* or *hereditary factors*. Intelligent parents tend to have intelligent children. The average I.Q. for children of professional fathers is 116; for unskilled labourers it is 95; identical twins have similar I.Q.s. However, *environmental factors* certainly have some influence and identical twins brought up apart show larger differences in I.Q. than those reared together. Intellectual stimulation from the home is important and may help to explain part of the difference between the children of labourers and professional men. A cultured background stimulates the child and provides maximum opportunity for the child's basic abilities to emerge. Children from better class homes tend to do better than those from families in the lower social groups. Homes of the latter tend to be more crowded, parents are less interested in their child's efforts, and there is less stimulation generally. Children from small families develop better intellectually than those from large ones. The effect of being one of a one or two child family, compared to a five or more child family, is to show a gain in reading age of 12 months by the age of 7.

SUBNORMALITY

Although people of I.Q. less than 70 are usually classified as *subnormal*, it is important to realize that such a classification can never be made simply on the results of a test, but depends on other factors, particularly personality and sociability. After all, in practice a person can only be subnormal in relation to his environment. He may be able to adapt normally to one environment but not to another.

Subnormals between I.Q. 50 and 70 (formerly known as feeble-minded) are part of the normal distribution of inherited intelligence. On the whole they come from families of below average intelligence. But those with I.Q.s below 50, the *severely subnormal*, tend to come from all social classes. This type of *subnormality* is often caused by single abnormal genes, by physical agents which damage the unborn child, such as *rubella* or *rhesus incompatibility*, or by brain injury or infection in childhood (see p. 172).

ASSESSING INTELLIGENCE IN A PATIENT

A good intelligence is generally associated with a wide vocabulary; conversely people with below average intelligence tend to have a limited vocabulary. It is important for nurses to recognize this association and make due allowance for it when explaining illness or treatment to a patient. Patients may be too frightened to say that they do not understand and, in consequence, may be made more fearful rather than reassured by the nurse's well-meant but incomprehensible explanation. It is just as important, however, not to 'talk down' to a patient.

Lastly it should be remembered that (statistically speaking) intelligence is inversely related to neurotic and behavioural disorders; that is, the lower the intelligence, the more frequent these become.

3

PERSONALITY

Some people are always optimistic and happy, others are gloomy and pessimistic. Some are always clean and tidy, and some less so. One person hates what another likes. We could continue such a list of contrasts almost indefinitely, for as many times as there are people in the world. No two people are exactly alike, not even identical twins, and the differences make up *personality*.

Personality describes the whole person, his attitudes, moods, characteristic behaviour, the way he parts his hair, the type of girl-friend he has, the books he likes, his height, and so on. Personality is not accidental. It is determined by both heredity and environment, just as height depends partly on the height of parents and ancestors and partly on proper nourishment during the growth period. Family and cultural influences account for many of the differences between families and races. Early childhood experiences of achieving satisfaction of needs, especially those connected with parents or other important adults, influence the way in which adult desires and needs are satisfied. But children brought up under the same roof may differ widely from one another. One child may develop into a *psychopathic personality*, selfish and egocentric, another may become obsessional and over-concerned about people, while a third may be happy and carefree, able to give and receive affection equally. These differences are probably due to hereditary factors.

Personality can be divided, rather artificially, into *temperament* and *character*.

Temperament describes someone's characteristic mood.

Character describes a person's qualities, his attitudes and behaviour.

Nations and races often differ widely in character. Even in our own country there are differences between those living in different regions. Compared with Americans, English people are often stand-offish and difficult to get to know. Margaret Mead, the anthropologist, found big differences of character between neighbouring tribes in New Guinea, all of whom are probably descended from the same stock. In one tribe men and women have passive, meek characters, quite the opposite of the aggressive characteristics of the people of a neighbouring tribe. In a third tribe the men are 'effeminate', while their women folk are domineering and carry out what we would regard as the masculine role. These differences of character seem to be closely related to the way each tribe brings up and treats its children, and to the different parts played by men and women in each tribe.

We have already emphasized that the infant is born largely unformed, ready to be moulded by his environment. Society, acting at first through the family, keeps him alive and teaches him its values, beliefs, accepted patterns of behaviour, and customs accumulated from the past that make up *culture*. Culture varies from one society to the next, and a man from one culture inevitably differs in many ways from a man of another. Behaviour which is regarded as abnormal or undesirable in one society may be acceptable or even thought to be desirable in another. But for a child to become a developed human being as we understand the term, he must be moulded by his culture and stimulated by other human beings. Children who have been abandoned in the wilds in infancy have occasionally survived and been found years later. Such creatures have aptly been described as 'wolf children'. They cannot speak, and they behave like wild animals rather than humans. They have been deprived of the normal contact and stimulation that are necessary to normal development.

Children who are born with one or more of their senses seriously impaired—for instance, blind or deaf children—may also have developmental difficulties unless special efforts are made to establish human communication, as happened with Helen Keller.

We live in a time of rapid change. Customs and beliefs constantly change, and there is often a lack of any sense of permanence or stability in our society. In a traditional or primitive society where change is infinitely slow, customs are long-standing and fixed. Everyone knows his position and what is expected of him. In a constantly changing society customs are not so fixed. People are uncertain of their position and therefore feel insecure. As a result they may conform excessively to the patterns of behaviour set by their neighbours. Such conformity results in rigidity and unadaptability. This may lead to disorganization and disruption of personality and behaviour.

ABNORMAL BEHAVIOUR AND SOCIETY

Behaviour which is regarded as abnormal in one society may be acceptable in another; and even in the same society certain forms of behaviour may be acceptable to one generation but not to the following ones. Homosexuality was acceptable to the ancient Greeks, but much less so to us. Transvestites (see p. 118) are given psychiatric treatment in our society, but in some tribal societies it is perfectly acceptable for men to take on the role and dress of women. Anyone in our country today who sees visions or hears messages from God, is usually considered to be in need of medical treatment. Yet not so long ago such experiences were readily accepted as coming from supernatural sources. Even today in certain tribes, witch-doctors need to have hallucinations in order to be successful. To increase the intensity of their experiences they indulge in fasting or drug-taking. Yet no one believes that these witch-doctors are mad, for they are astute and fully in touch with what is happening around them. Behaviour or experience can only be judged against the framework of the cultural environment, and in relation to the whole personality. Mental disorder occurs in all societies, although symptoms vary with the culture. Invariably the personality of anyone mentally ill shows signs of distintegration. Society is liable to make scapegoats of some of its members. The senile, eccentric and mentally ill, particularly if female, were persecuted and burnt as witches in their thousands throughout Europe and America during the 15th, 16th and 17th centuries.

During the next two centuries 'masturbators' were sought out and 'treated'. In some families today one member acts as the scapegoat and may be regarded as mentally ill. Ronald Laing, among others, has written much about this particular problem.

EFFECTS OF DIFFERENT SOCIAL CONDITIONS ON BEHAVIOUR

Knowledge of a man's character enables his behaviour to be roughly predictable under certain circumstances. He may be very brave, and you can be pretty certain how he will behave in a fight. But alter the environment and change the situation from a physical to a moral one. Now the brave man may well become a coward. He may have won a V.C. on the battlefield, but he is too frightened of his boss to ask him for a rise in pay or an extra day's holiday.

A group of people in any situation always throws up a leader. A leader must possess certain qualities of intelligence, self-confidence and so on, but under different conditions and circumstances, different people emerge as leaders. Another place in which differences of behaviour under different circumstances have been studied is in the classroom. It has been shown that children may cheat in certain situations but not in others. In all these cases behaviour is clearly the result of personality interacting with different social environments.

A person's behaviour also varies with the people he is with. This depends partly on the social position, partly on the personality of the other person, and on many other things too. Your attitude towards the hospital kitchen-maid is quite different from your attitude towards the matron. You may become gay and abandoned when with a joyful person, or morose and bored with a gloomy one. If you are a forceful personality you may clash with an equally domineering one. And you may quickly tire of the company of someone whose interests differ widely from your own.

We all play many roles. A man may be a bank manager, husband, father, son, member of a golf club, justice of the peace, to list a few of his roles. He may behave very differently in each of these groups and situations, and his behaviour in one role may clash with his behaviour in another. He may be a ruthless and unscrupulous businessman and a devout churchgoer.

The size of a group also influences the behaviour of its members. Small groups work together better than large ones. The more the group members like each other, the more *cohesive* is the group; and the more cohesive the group, the greater the *conformity* of its members towards the 'group average'. On the other hand, members of a cohesive group derive a feeling of security from 'belonging' to the group, which encourages individuality. Cohesion is also increased if the group feels itself threatened by outsiders, a fact well known to the political leaders of small parties.

Internal dissension, and even the presence of a single disgruntled member, weaken and split the group. This effect can sometimes be seen in the hospital wards. A single bored or unhappy nurse may upset the atmosphere of the whole ward. An insecure ward sister makes life difficult for nurses and patients alike. And almost always an unhappy ward is inefficient.

CLASSIFYING AND MEASURING PERSONALITY

Personality can be described in terms of types or traits. The ancient Greeks divided people into four types, depending upon which of four humours predominated. The predominance of black bile produced a melancholic type, pessimistic and moody. An excess of yellow bile was related to a choleric type, irritable and active. The sanguine man possessed an excess of blood and was optimistic and outgoing. Lastly, the phlegmatic man, with an excess of phlegm, was sluggish and rather apathetic.

We no longer think of humours, but is only a few years since people were divided into 'endocrine types'. Thus the 'thyroid' personality, who was supposed to have a high level of circulating thyroid hormone, was highly strung and excitable. The 'adrenal' type was driving and ambitious. Hormones certainly influence behaviour and mood, but few people now believe that personality can be satisfactorily classified in terms of hormones.

The relationship between a man's physical build and his temperament has long been recognized. In recent times Kretschmer tried to crystallize this belief. He noticed that his *schizophrenic* patients tended to be *asthenic*, lean, flat chested, with narrow shoulders, while the *manic-depressive* patients were shorter and rounder, or *pyknic* (like John Bull). He extended his study to normal people, and found that those with an asthenic build tended to be emotionally cold, unsociable and introspective, resembling in minor form the schizophrenic personality. Conversely, those of *pyknic* build tended to be sociable and energetic, moody, alternating between depression and happiness, like manic-depressive patients. Eventually he classified everyone into one of three types; the *asthenic*, with a *schizoid* personality; the *pyknic*, with a *cyclothymic* personality; and an intermediate type which he called *athletic*. (He also included a fourth type, the *displastic*, for those who did not fit into any of the first three types.)

Sheldon has tried to make this classification more objective. He took photographs of the nude body from three angles, from which he made certain measurements. Each person is rated on a seven-point scale, each of three *somatotype* components, *ectomorphy*, *endomorphy* and *mesomorphy*. (These correspond to Kretschmer's pyknic, asthenic and athletic respectively.) Thus, an extreme ectomorph is expressed as *117*, an extreme *endomorph* as *711*, and an extreme *mesomorph* as *171*. In practice most people have somatotypes somewhere between these extremes. Sheldon describes a *viscerotonic* personality linked with endomorphy, a *cerebrotonic* personality linked with ectomorphy, and a *somatotonic* personality linked with mesomorphy.

The terms *introvert* and *extravert* were first used by Carl Jung to describe personality. An extravert is sociable, outgoing, a man of action rather than thought, a 'feely' rather than a 'thinky'. The introvert, on the other hand, is much more concerned with his own inner world.

Jung's views were supported by Eysenck's studies. Studying a large number of healthy and neurotic soldiers, and submitting his data to factorial analysis, he found two orthogonal bipolar dimensions of personality: these he named extraversion–introversion, and neuroticism–stability. The introvert was likely to be unsociable and cautious and if neurotic to develop anxiety or reactive depression. The extravert, on the other hand, was outgoing, and if neurotic was likely to develop hysterical symptoms. Eysenck later claimed a third dimension, psychoticism. Eysenck went on to link up his work with some of Pavlov's ideas. He suggested that extraversion was characterized by cortical inhibition, introversion by excitation. In general, experimental work has confirmed his views.

A rather different type of classification originated from Freud. Freud noted that young children respond with pleasure to stimulation of virtually any part of their bodies, sometimes so intensely as to suggest a reaction akin to sexual pleasure. He postulated the existence of certain erotogenic zones or areas, stimulation of which gave particular pleasure in certain stages of development: the mouth region for the first 18 months, the anus for the next two years, and then the genital organs. The development of a normal personality entailed passing through these phases. Disappointments and frustrations might cause the child to become 'fixated' at that level of development, and this subsequently would determine his personality characteristics. Thus the oral type is a dependent type expecting to be looked after. The anal character is orderly, parsimonious and obstinate. Toilet training is given much credit for producing this type of character. Those fixated at the phallic stage are likely to be rather narcissistic, ambitious and exhibitionistic.

Personality traits are characteristics which can be measured by objective personality tests. In the U.S.A. Cattell, using factor analysis, has searched for the source traits, which he regards as the fundamental structure of personality. He sees a trait as a 'mental structure', which is regularly and consistently present. He has isolated 16 primary factors, including out-going–reserved, tense–relaxed, self-sufficient–group dependent, con-scientious–expedient, suspicious–trusting, venturesome–shy. In practice, clinical psychiatrists find it convenient to describe a personality in rather looser terms: *obsessive, hysterical, schizoid, paranoid, anxious, cyclothymic, depressive.*

The *obsessive* personality is excessively conscientious, tidy, pedantic, punctual and reliable. He tends to check whatever he does. He does not like change, and is upset by any alteration of his routine. He likes to feel he is in complete control of himself and his world. He keeps his emotions well under control, and rarely loses his temper. His sense of humour tends to be limited. Some obsessive personalities go to the opposite extreme in certain respects; they may be meticulous about everything except being punctual, and they may turn up hours late for their appointments. Or they may be extraordinarily untidy at home, although their office and their work are excessively neat and tidy. It seems that they must either control their environment completely, or make no attempt at all; no compromise is possible.

To interview a really obsessive patient is to understand clearly his con-flict between obedience and defiance: he constantly tries to control the interview, repeatedly glances at his watch, pulls out enormous lists of notes which he asks to read, and creates considerable boredom and irrita-tion in the interviewer.

The *hysterical* personality is very different. She needs to feel she is the centre of the stage. She seems to be continually playing a part, and con-tinually changing her personality. In many ways she is like a small child, making excessive demands and exhausting those around her. Emotional scenes and dramas are occurring constantly. She falls in love, but no one lives up to her ideals and everyone fails her. She is incapable of experienc-ing any real depths of emotion, yet she goes from one extreme to another. A small slight will be magnified into a deadly insult; a thoughtless word will become a declaration of love, or evidence that she is no longer loved, and so on. The most exhausting scenes will be forgotten as quickly as they began, and she will be hurt when others cannot forget or forgive so easily. The hysterical personality is perhaps nearest to what the psychoanalysts call an oral character. She is looking for an ideal parent figure on whom she can depend. Difficult and childlike in behaviour as these patients may be at times, they are never dull and they can be extremely stimulating for the interviewer. It is perhaps not unexpected that hysterical personalities and obsessional personalities are attracted to one another.

The *schizoid* personality is shy, withdrawn and 'shut in'. He is emo-tionally cold and is unable to mix and form deep friendships. Often he is eccentric in his habits and leads a life of his own, apart from other people.

33

The *paranoid* personality is suspicious of everyone. He is touchy, and lacks a sense of humour. He has an inflated idea of his own abilities and is difficult to work with, being rigid and unadaptable. He has few friends.

The *anxious* personality is a lifelong worrier, always anticipating the worst, and doubting to the last. His sympathetic nervous system is over-reactive, and bodily symptoms are liable to occur when he is emotionally upset.

The *cyclothymic personality* is prone to alternating moods of elation and gloom, often without obvious cause.

The *depressive* personality is pessimistic, lacking in zest and energy, and afraid to allow his potentials fully to develop.

The usefulness of these clinical descriptions lies in the fact that when people break down, they usually do so in characteristic ways that reflect their personality structure.

PERSONALITY TESTS. '*Paper and Pencil*' *questionnaires* can sometimes be useful, but they have disadvantages. Answers may reflect what people like to think they are rather than what they really are, and it is difficult to exclude deliberate untruths. Examples of the type of question asked are:

Do you feel that people look at you when you enter a crowded room? .   .   .   .   Yes or No.
Do you express your feelings openly when upset by someone? .   .   .   .   Yes or No.
Do you enjoy going to parties?   .   .   .   Yes or No.

Projective tests include the *Rorschach* and *thematic apperception tests*. The individual is presented with a stimulus which has no particular meaning or structure, and into which he 'projects' his own feelings and experiences. Thereby he reveals different aspects of his personality.

The *Rorschach test* consists of ten cards containing ink-blots. The subject describes what he sees in each. These, and his emotional reactions to the ink blots, are then scored and interpreted. There has been much criticism of the reliability of this test. Subjective factors undoubtedly affect the result, but good results are obtained by skilled and experienced psychologists.

The *thematic apperception test* consists of a series of pictures without obvious meaning. The subject is asked to say what the picture represents. He may identify himself with various characters, and reveal information about himself which, in the case of a patient, may be useful in psychotherapy.

MENTAL MECHANISMS

In psychoanalytical terms, the ego is that part of the psyche which is adapting constantly to the pressures of the instincts (id), the conscience (super ego) and external reality. Defence mechanisms are employed by the ego to maintain a satisfactory adaptation. The same mechanisms are used by normal, neurotic, and psychotic people, but obviously there is likely to be a much greater distortion of reality in psychotic illness. (See p. 85.) Different personalities tend to differ in the mechanisms they habitually employ. All these mechanisms are considered to be 'unconscious'.

Repression underlies all the defence mechanisms. Through repression the ego prevents all unbearable wishes, feelings and impulses from reaching consciousness. A simple example of repression is 'forgetting' an unpleasant appointment. Repression needs to be distinguished from *suppression*, which is a conscious attempt to control unacceptable ideas or impulses, and denial. A man dying of terminal carcinoma may deny he is ill and plan his holiday for next year. A wife, suddenly bereaved, will deny her husband is dead.

Reaction formation. An unacceptable attitude is prevented from becoming conscious by the adoption of the opposite attitude. A man with strong homosexual leanings becomes vitriolic and intolerant to homosexuals.

Displacement. This is a common mechanism in everyday life. Feelings are displaced from some person who is desired or feared on to someone or something else less dangerous. The ward sister, criticized by her superior, may displace her aggressive feelings on to one of her nurses and give her a severe dressing down. The nurse in turn perhaps vents her anger on her boy friend.

Transference, the relationship which springs up between doctor and patient and nurse and patient, is based upon displacement, the patient displacing unconscious emotions and attitudes of earlier childhood relationships onto the doctor or nurse. Similar displacement mechanisms are involved in *counter transference,* the unconscious emotional attitude of the doctor and nurse towards their patient.

Identification or introjection. Through this mechanism a person identifies with, and models himself upon, another person. It is regarded as an important factor in the development of a child's personality, and psychosexual identity. It is made use of in behaviour therapy (modelling). Identification is also a means by which unacceptable impulses are made acceptable. For instance, a man with strong sadistic wishes identifies with a sadistic, powerful person.

Projection. Unacceptable feelings are not only repressed but attributed to, i.e. projected onto, someone else. A woman projects her unacceptable sexual feelings for another man onto him, and believes that he is constantly trying to seduce her. Although common enough in children, adult projection usually entails considerable distortion of reality.

Substitution. Unacceptable impulses are switched into acceptable activities. Murderous rage is used up in punching a pillow or chopping down a tree.

Sublimation. Unacceptable sexual and aggressive drives are, by this mechanism, directed into socially acceptable channels. Freud considered that civilizations arose through the sublimation of sexual instincts.

4

MATURATION

Maturation is development rather than growth. A new-born child has legs, but cannot use them for walking; if he is premature he may even be unable to suck. At one year old, though he may be able to take a few steps on his own, he will not be able to talk, and he will still be wet at night. A child of five may 'fall in love', but his feelings and behaviour will be quite unlike those of an adult who has fallen in love, and he will certainly not be capable of adult sexual behaviour.

Maturation occurs progressively. A child who has had a normal full-term delivery can suck, swallow, breathe and carry out functions that are essential for life and growth. This is because his central nervous system, as well as the organs concerned, has matured and developed its organizations sufficiently for these actions to be possible. After birth, the nervous system continues to mature, and there is a corresponding orderly growth of behaviour. Sitting up, standing, walking, sphincter control, language and sexual behaviour can occur only when the nervous system is sufficiently mature to organize them. Until the appropriate stage of maturity has been reached, these things will not be possible, no matter how strong the demand from the environment. Thus, however much a mother wants her child to talk, walk or be dry, and however hard she tries to persuade him in these matters, she will not be successful until his nervous system is sufficiently developed to cope with them. Since there is an enormous amount of individual variation, one child will learn these things much more quickly than another.

Even when the nervous system is sufficiently mature to learn certain modes of behaviour, these may not in fact occur unless there is suitable stimulation from the environment. No matter how mature is his nervous system, a child will not learn Greek unless someone teaches him. For the same reason some people continue to wet their beds throughout their lives simply because they were never taught sphincter control.

There is a rough level of maturity for each age. But it is very rough, because normal individuals can differ so widely from each other.

Infants and young children have characteristic brain-waves, as recorded by *electroencephalogram*. These brain-waves are thought to reflect the still immature organization of the brain. As the child grows older, the 'immature' waves tend to die out, and they only appear under special conditions. It is interesting to note that in some adults, particularly *psychopaths*, this immature type of record may persist. It is possible that the impulsive, egocentric and childlike behaviour of psychopaths may be related to the lack of maturation of the brain.

As we grow older maturation changes into rigidity. Learning and adaptability become progressively more difficult and eventually cease with the onset of senility.

5

FAMILY

A parent can be rejecting, over-protective, ambivalent or, like the average, a 'mixture'. A totally rejecting parent is unusual, at the most probably less than 1 per cent of the population. The rejected child represents something unacceptable to one or both parents. More common is over-protection. A child may be over-protected for many reasons; because of a parent's own sense of insecurity, as over-compensation for guilt aroused by feelings of rejection, when the child is born after the death or serious illness of a sibling, or a series of miscarriages, or because one parent is using the child to compensate for marital dissatisfactions.

Ambivalent maternal emotions during pregnancy and for a short time after delivery are common. Positive feelings of love and protection rapidly build up in most mothers when they see and hold their infants. But ambivalent feelings sometimes remain strong, resulting in over-protection alternating with rejection, or what is known as *double bind*. This describes a situation between two people, closely involved with one another, where one person gives conflicting contradictory signals to the other. For instance, a mother will hold out her arms to her son and say, 'Come and give me a kiss', but in such a tone of voice and with such a hostile look that the child does not know what action to take. The child may be rewarded and loved only when he succeeds and pleases, and is scolded or ignored when he fails to match up to parental expectations. Thus he quickly comes to feel that he is loved not for what or who he is, but only for what he achieves. He may rebel and become unmanageable at home. Or he may inhibit his deeper emotions, particularly those concerning aggression, and become an excessively hardworking 'model' child. Thus his personality develops.

THE BATTERED BABY SYNDROME

At least 3000 infants and children are injured or seriously deprived each year in the U.K., and at least 40 of these infants die. The child who is battered is usually between a few weeks and 3 years old, although he can be much older. Violence tends to be episodic and occurs when one or both parents become tried beyond their endurance by the crying or the negativism of the child. The mortality rate among battered babies is substantial, and a high proportion of the survivors are brain damaged or permanently crippled.

Battering parents come from all social classes. They were commonly abused themselves as children, and perhaps learnt at an early age to react aggressively to difficulties and tension. They tend to be inadequate personalities, unable to tolerate their child's fractious behaviour without resorting to violence. Sometimes a battering parent is psychotic, has postpartum depression or is of subnormal intelligence (although subnormality bears no direct relationship to battering). But only about 5 per cent are ill in the strict psychiatric sense. If a parent batters his first-born child, the risk of further children being battered is very high.

Practitioners are often reluctant to diagnose the 'battered baby syndrome', preferring to overlook the possibility. Any suspicion, any delay in bringing the baby for treatment of injuries, twist injuries of the joints, or multiple scattered injuries, should be investigated by a complete skeletal X-ray examination.

A Care and Protection Order may be needed if a child is thought to be at risk. Needless to say, as the American psychiatrist Kempe has reiterated: 'Criminal penalties for battering parents are absolutely useless'.

SOCIAL AND LIVING CONDITIONS

Social conditions contribute to parental reactions, and influence the way children develop. Overcrowding increases after each child, and is particularly likely to effect adversely the illegitimate child. Children may encounter hostile neighbours and be frightened to go alone into streets and playground. Racial tensions may grow and cause anxiety among coloured children.

Problem families exist in every large urban area, unable to fend for themselves in the manner demanded by society. They may be evicted from their homes for non-payment of rent. If their home is broken up, children are uprooted from their schools, taken from teachers and other trusted people on whom they have come to depend. Or parents may be sent to prison for thieving and their children put into care and protection. It is important to recognize that children can have important relationships outside their families which will be shattered if the family is split or moved, sometimes with serious consequences for the child.

It is often difficult for immature and anxious parents to cope with social and cultural pressures, particularly when they move into new and unfamiliar areas, next to people of different social backgrounds. Anxious parents fear their child showing them up, and try to discipline him into behaving 'properly'. The child may react angrily to his parents' sense of shame and inferiority, thus setting up a vicious circle. Parents with fragile psychological defences are liable to break down under such social pressures.

And like their children they then regress in behaviour. Social pressures of this kind on parents are likely to be greater if their children are handicapped, and are singled out for attention by neighbours.

Faced with such a situation a child finds the pressures increasingly hard to tolerate and may gradually become near-psychotic in behaviour. Sooner or later he will have to be removed from this disrupting environment. Social and cultural pressures will have combined to destroy, perhaps permanently, the bond between parents and child.

6

DEVELOPMENT

There is no real evidence showing that a breast-fed infant develops more satisfactorily than a bottle-fed infant. Fifty years ago breast-feeding was definitely preferable because less was known about the nutritional needs of infants and also because bottle-feeding was unhygienic. But today, from the point of view of hygiene and nutrition, bottle-feeding is as satisfactory as breast-feeding. But tactile stimulation does seem to be important, and the amount of handling a child receives is probably much more important than how he is fed. Emotional difficulties and tensions in his mother may be transmitted to the child through the way he is handled.

The infant needs food and comfort. When he is satisfied he feels pleasure. The satisfaction becomes associated with his mother and other people who satisfy his needs. Gradually, by a sort of conditioning process, the mother herself becomes a need; now the infant feels pleasure when she is with him and handling him. He feels unrest when she is absent.

The infant's relaxed contented state is satisfying to the mother, but even more so is the child's smiling. The feedback from the child to its mother is important. Mother needs to feel and see her child responding to her, smiling at her, moulding his body to hers and so on. The screaming child who refuses to eat, usually in response to tensions from her, increases her anxiety. The autistic child creates coldness in his mother. Smiling develops at about six weeks. (Smiling begins later in prematurely born infants, indicating that internal growth factors are more important than environmental.) At first the smile is merely a reflex response on the part of a *satisfied* infant to a human face. Until he is four or five months old he is probably incapable of recognizing anyone. Certainly the child does not begin to form his first important attachment or bond with his parents or parent substitute until about six months of age. The practical importance of this is that during these first few months it probably does not matter who, or how many people, look after the child provided his needs are satisfied. However, once memory begins to develop and the child can recognize his mother as a person who satisfies his needs, her presence does become important for his development. From five or six months onwards he may show signs of anxiety when she is away. Such anxiety is likely to be greater in a child whose early needs were not fully satisfied, either because of circumstances or because of emotional difficulties in his mother. Such a child may quickly become restless when his mother is absent and he may be excessively demanding of her attentions. Any lengthy separation from his mother may result in considerable and prolonged anxiety which may interfere with his development. (We discuss the effects of 'maternal deprivation' on p. 46.) It is important to recognize that organic factors such as damage in utero or some minor injury at birth insufficient to cause cerebral palsy but sufficient to cause sensory deficiencies may also interfere with the child's development.

In general, it seems likely that the way in which a child's needs are satisfied in his early years largely determines how he will deal with his needs when he is an adult. Discomfort and anxiety resulting from continually unsatisfied needs may cause difficulties later, particularly in human relationships. However, this does not mean that the infant's every wish should be instantly met, or that his mother should subordinate completely her own feelings and needs to those of her child. Excessive spoiling of a child may cause just as much trouble later as deprivation, for it may result in the *pleasure principle* being carried on into adult life.

The *pleasure principle* describes how the new-born child expects his every need to be instantly satisfied. The infant is at first not aware of any differentiation between himself and the outside world. The breast or bottle, when he is hungry and is fed, becomes part of himself. But gradually he comes to distinguish objects and beings external to himself, and sooner or later he comes to recognize that other people also have needs. He learns that these needs sometimes conflict with his own. And he learns that it is sometimes necessary to postpone the gratification of his needs, otherwise he may incur the disapproval of his mother or some other important person in his life. And the fact that he may lose the affection of such people is upsetting. This is the beginning of the *reality principle*, and from now on the child realizes increasingly that he must adapt his needs to those of others, and that he can no longer expect always to have his own way.

From about two years onwards *repression* (see p. 35) begins to operate increasingly, preventing wholly unacceptable impulses and wishes from coming into consciousness. This is the beginning of acceptable social behaviour. But the child at this stage behaves and controls his impulses because he knows he may be punished if he does what he wants. If he knows he will certainly not be caught, then he may steal a box of sweets or do anything else that attracts him. A code of behaviour based on such an equilibrium of pleasure and reality will certainly cause difficulties if carried into adult life.

Most of us behave in accordance with a higher principle, that of *conscience*. This is a moral sense involving real considerations for the needs of others. A conscience develops in most children around the age of seven or eight years as a result of adopting and incorporating the attitudes, beliefs and customs of people who are loved and admired. Such people are parents, teachers, close friends, and so on. A secure, happy child who loves and admires his parents has no difficulty in *identifying* (see p. 35) himself with what he sees to be their good qualities, for he feels that he must live up to their high standards. But an insecure child, perhaps without a mother, may not be able to do this and conscience may only form much later or not at all. Defective learning of this type, due to deprivation, is probably responsible for some *psychopaths* who lack a moral sense and who are unable to control their impulses.

The formation of a conscience may also be delayed or affected if a child is excessively pampered or spoilt. Then the child or adult may continue to operate on the pleasure principle, even though such a person may himself suffer from his behaviour. It seems that there may be a *critical period* for the development of a conscience, and that if this is missed for any reason, subsequent development is very slow and perhaps always defective to some degree.

As the infant's *memory* develops, so does his *self-awareness*. He begins to distinguish himself from his outside world. Gradually he learns to recognize his hands, arms, legs and feet, and so on, as part of himself and memory adds permanence to his state of identity. As sensation and motor co-ordination grow, with maturation of the central nervous system, so self-awareness grows and is probably well developed by between two and three years old.

His growing sense of identity and his increasing agility lead, by the end of the first year of life, to his trying increasingly to assert his independence. Struggles may develop between mother and child at this time, and reach a peak around eighteen months to two years. He becomes obstinate and negativistic and seems to take pleasure in refusing to co-operate or do what he is asked. Constant scenes and struggles may occur at meal-times or when he is put to bed. He refuses to use his pot, but almost immediately dirties himself or makes a puddle on the floor or wets the bed. All too easily a vicious circle may build up; his mother loses her sense of proportion and matters get completely out of hand. Some firmness and discipline is essential, but too harsh or punitive an attitude may inhibit his development and result in his becoming too conforming and docile. Provided the child is allowed a reasonable amount of self-expression and is not over-suppressed and over-protected, he will gradually become more constructive and co-operative. This positive process is usually increased by mixing and playing with other children.

For the first three years the child's mother is usually the most important figure and influence in his life. He will come to recognize his father during the first year, but it is not until later, around the third or fourth year, that he really begins to take notice of him and imitate his ways. If the child is a boy he may begin to show signs of jealousy and try to monopolize his mother's attention. A girl, on the other hand, may try to compete with her mother for her father's affection. This family triangle was depicted by Sophocles two thousand years ago in Oedipus Rex. Freud borrowed from the title and described this 'normal' phase of development under the term *Oedipus complex*. Although many children do show some jealousy to the parent of the same sex, and openly favour the other, it is doubtful whether this situation always occurs in our present-day society, and it is certainly unknown in some cultures. Its existence probably depends to some extent on the family's attitude to childhood sexual behaviour. The more this is frowned upon, the more likely are *Oedipus* feelings to emerge.

In any case these feelings form only a small part of the relationship that exists between the child and his father. Just as a girl identifies herself with her mother and becomes increasingly feminine, so a boy needs to identify himself with his father and acquire his masculine ways. These processes of identification interact with constitutional factors. In general, boys tend to be more aggressive than girls; and this characteristic, under the influence of the male sex hormones, increases after puberty.

SIBLING RIVALRY

Much has been written about the effect on a child of a new baby in the family. So far as young children are concerned signs of jealousy towards the new baby are 'normal'. Jealousy is likely to be particularly obvious in children who had a very close relationship with their mothers; first-born children are therefore likely to be more affected than later born. The jealous child feels he will lose the affection of his parents, and it is important for parents to recognize and understand this. If the child feels particularly insecure and rejected (this will depend largely upon his earlier experiences) he may *regress* in behaviour. He then starts to behave as he did when younger. For instance, having been dry he may start to be dirty, refuse to eat properly, demand a bottle instead of a cup, or revert to 'baby talk'. A wise mother prepares the child for the new baby's arrival and lets him share in the preparations. And subsequently, within limits, she lets him help look after the baby, and is tolerant about his difficult behaviour.

The mixed feelings of a child towards his new-born brother or sister are often quite apparent. He will rock the cot or pat the baby's head, at first in play, but gradually becoming increasingly rough until he is virtually attacking the infant. He may be very friendly towards the baby as long as he gets on well with his mother, but in a moment when he is angry with his mother, he may attack the baby. With time and parental understanding these jealousies subside.

The position of a child in the family may influence his development and his personality. First-born children are often particularly close to their mothers and, perhaps because they receive more attention than those born later, they tend to be more advanced in their development. Statistically they are more intelligent in terms of I.Q. than those born later. Sometimes, however, the oldest of a large family may be restricted by the activities of the younger children and may be called upon to assume an excessive amount of responsibility. The youngest child—particularly if there is a large gap between him and the next child—and the only child are both liable to be spoilt and over-mothered and kept emotionally younger than their years.

CHILDHOOD HABITS

Certain forms of behaviour are so common in younger children that they can be regarded as normal, although they may worry parents. Almost all children, for instance, suck their thumbs at some time. They derive considerable satisfaction from this. Usually the habit stops before the age of about four years, but sometimes it persists and may occasionally give rise to orthodontic troubles, although there is no need to worry about this until the second teeth are through. Night terrors, when the child is terrified although awake, occur most often between two and three years. Head banging, hair-pulling, and masturbation may come and go. Nail-biting usually begins at about three or four years and may continue on and off for many years. 8 per cent of social class 1 and 13 per cent of social class 5 are bad nail biters still at the age of seven. Tics and habit spasms are also common and usually disappear quickly if ignored.

Neurotic disorders such as phobias, obsessions and general unhappiness of mood are not uncommon. They do of course cause misery not only to the child but to his family, and may interfere with his progress at school, but in themselves they have no clear significance for the development of later psychiatric disorder. On the other hand, antisocial behaviour in childhood is significant. Children who are persistently antisocial in behaviour are likely to grow worse after puberty and to become delinquent. In addition, they have more marital difficulties, worse work records, poorer social relationships, more general psychiatric illness and poorer physical health.

EMOTIONAL DEPRIVATION

Emotional deprivation is all too readily equated with maternal deprivation, which is still a controversial subject. Interest in maternal deprivation developed in the mid-1930s, and in 1951 John Bowlby summarized all published works in a report to the World Health Organization. He concluded that 'Maternal love in infancy is as important for mental health as are vitamins and proteins for physical health', and that 'prolonged deprivation of the young child of maternal care may have grave and far reaching effects on his character, and so on the whole of his future life'. A child needs 'a warm intimate and continuous relationship with his mother in which both find satisfaction and enjoyment'. Bowlby severely criticized the institutional care of children, including the way they were looked after in hospitals. His work has stimulated much research, both human and a variety of animal studies (which cannot easily be compared with humans as is sometimes done rather naïvely). Some of his conclusions were widely misinterpreted. Mothers were expected to spend 24 hours a day with their children. Mother love was elevated to almost mystical heights. Working mothers were castigated, and so were nurses and crèches.

Until the age of about six months, a child does not begin to form a bond with his mother or substitute figure. Any sizeable break in the child's relationship with his mother, particularly between the ages of six months and five years, may adversely affect his development, particularly his later ability to socialize with other people. For instance, Bowlby's original study of 44 thieves suggested that psychopathy was particularly likely to be related to frequent changes of mother figures during the first two years. Certainly a *failure to form bonds* in the first three years, due to emotional deprivation is liable to lead to 'affectionless psychopathy' later. On the other hand, *disruption of bonds* already forged characteristically produces acute distress in the child. But many factors are involved, and it is as well to keep a sense of proportion and to realize that many young children are separated from their mothers for long periods at a time and do not appear to suffer damage. Constitutional factors, the child's sense of security at the time of separation, who looks after him in place of his mother, knowledge of the future, and so on, are all important in this respect. Although John Bowlby's main work has been concerned with the adverse effect of a long separation of the child from his mother, he has also pointed out that maternal deprivation can arise when the child's mother is unable to give him all the loving care he needs because of her own emotional difficulties. But the harmful effects of separation have probably been exaggerated and have led to unnecessary anxiety on the part of many parents. On the other hand, a high proportion of juvenile delinquents and people with psychopathic personalities do come from broken homes that are lacking in affection, or they have been separated from their mothers in early childhood. A child whose parents constantly row or separate is less likely to feel the security which is so important if he is to identify himself with his parents, and acquire social and moral standards. Often the child becomes a pawn in the parents' quarrels, being used by the mother or father in turn to score off the other; the child quickly learns to use this situation for his own ends for he senses a basic lack of affection for him in such parents. Mothers may encourage their daughters to fear men and to regard anything to do with sex as nasty; thus they may perpetuate their own sexual difficulties in their daughters.

Contrasting with maternal deprivation is over-mothering, which may have equally harmful effects. In the U.S.A., over-mothering is sometimes known as *momism*. Momism is estimated to have cost the American Armed Forces more casualties than resulted from enemy action. The egocentric, immature, dependent personality that may result from momism is unable to adapt quickly or easily to new situations. It is essential that children should be exposed to a reasonable amount of stress from the time they are born, in order that adaptive mechanisms, both physiological and psychological, can develop.

There are many reasons for parents' abnormal attitudes towards their children, some of which have already been mentioned. The mother's attitude to her child usually relates closely to her relationship with her husband, and on whether the child was wanted. The child may have been conceived after a long period of sterility or been born after all the other children had grown up. Or the child may have been very ill and thus aroused persistent anxiety in his parents. Both parents may over-protect or reject the child because of problems in their own childhood. Or the parents may be unhappily married and compensate for their unhappiness through the child. In some instances over-protection may in fact be a compensation for underlying guilt and rejection of the child. Both parents may over-protect or reject the child because of problems in their own childhood. The father may resent bitterly the arrival of a baby and see him as a rival; not only may he reject the child but there may also be gross neglect or actual cruelty. If separated, both parents may use the child as a means of revenge through custody proceedings.

Bowlby believes the maternal bond with the child to be of special quality. This is disputed by many people and indeed there seems no good reason to suppose that it has any special quality, although it may be expected to be stronger because the mother sees most of the child.

There is evidence that women who feel a need to go out to work and do so are psychologically healthier as a result, and able to be more loving towards their children. There is no evidence that working mothers, provided they make satisfactory arrangements for their children's care, create extra psychological strains in their families. A clear-cut relationship exists between childhood disorders and an unhappy atmosphere at home. There is a strong chance that a child whose parents are constantly bickering will develop antisocial aggressive behaviour, or even become delinquent. From a forensic point of view, it is important to recognize that a child charged with some delinquent act is likely to repeat the offence if he returns to an unhappy home. It is better to send the child to a good institution, or for the family to split up and the child to be brought up by one parent, than for him to continue in this atmosphere. This has only been accepted by child care officers in the last few years. In the past, children were forced to remain in unsatisfactory homes because of child care officers' misunderstanding of Bowlby's earlier writings.

Consistent discipline is essential for the child. It does not matter much how the child is disciplined so long as discipline is consistent in its purpose. A child needs a framework in which to develop, outside which he knows he should not go. But excessive discipline may be harmful and result in later behaviour problems such as stealing, negativism, and outbursts of temper and destructiveness. It is always better to teach by example rather than by punishment. It is also important to appreciate that a child may be too young to understand why something he has done is wrong. Just as it is a waste of time to train a child to be dry before the central nervous system is developed at about eighteen months, so it does more harm than good to try to instil concepts or standards that the child cannot understand.

THE EFFECT OF PARENTAL ILLNESS

Chronic depression, psychopathy and neurosis in a parent are likely to produce psychiatric disorders in the child, especially of an antisocial nature. This is probably because neurotics tend to marry neurotics and because these disorders are associated with aggressive outbursts. On the other hand, schizophrenia in one parent doesn't seem to create psychiatric difficulties, mainly because the other partner is often stable and the home is not disturbed by quarrelling.

When both parents are mentally ill the family is likely to be disrupted and the chances of the child developing psychiatric disorder is high. About a third of the children seen in child guidance clinics have parents who are both ill mentally.

Physical illness in a parent of a chronic or recurrent type is twice as common among psychiatric children as among control groups. Psychiatrically disturbed children who continue to be mentally ill in later life are more likely to have experienced the death of one or more parent. Children between the ages of three and five are most vulnerable and likely to show long-term damage. The death of a parent in adolescence, particularly of the opposite sex, is liable to make the adolescent vulnerable to depression later on. Many factors of course are involved in a parent's death: length of time he was ill, whether by suicide, and particularly the reaction of the remaining partner.

ILLEGITIMATE CHILDREN

The rate of illegitimate births in Britain has risen sharply over the past 15 years. The illegitimate child, unless adopted at an early age, is at considerable disadvantage. He is usually the first-born child of a young mother, and is liable to be underweight at birth. When brought up by his natural parent, accommodation is likely to be poor and crowded. Compared to legitimate children the illegitimate child tends to be backward in ability and achievement at school, and to become maladjusted.

FOSTERED CHILDREN

Children without parents, or whose parents are unable to look after them, come under the care of the Children's Department of the local authority.

Whenever possible, particularly in infancy and in the pre-school period, children are boarded out in the care of foster parents, this being preferable to institutional care. Most children who are fostered are seriously deprived, and correspondingly disturbed emotionally. Foster parents usually require support and supervision from child care workers, responsible to the Child Care Officer.

Problems often arise in connection with the real parents. Many of them feel guilty towards their children and project hostile feelings on to the foster parents or the staff of the Children's Department. Such problems must be met with understanding by child workers.

ADOPTED CHILDREN

Adoption is probably the best form of *substitute* care for parentless children or those lacking a suitable home. Adopted children (statistically) develop better in every way than those in residential or foster care. The Adoption Act of 1958 has made it possible to dispense with a parent's consent to adoption if that parent has failed, without reasonable cause, to discharge his parental obligations.

Between 1 and 2 per cent of children are adopted, yet adopted children make up 5–13 per cent of referrals to child psychiatric clinics. The majority of these disturbed children have been adopted after the age of 6 months, a finding which emphasizes the adverse effect of early parental deprivation and the importance of children being placed with their adopted parents before 6 months.

Many of the couples who adopt are over 30 and have difficulty in adjusting to the infant's needs. Women often feel lingering shame over their inability to reproduce and this can increase their difficulties in disclosing to a child that he is adopted. Adoption societies carefully vet the reasons and personalities of couples wanting to adopt, for it is important that parents should face their conflicts and difficulties over the child honestly and frankly.

If the adopted child later becomes unhappy and disturbed, parents may refuse to see themselves as responsible, and will blame the child's heredity, his 'over-sexed' real parents, and so on.

Most of the additional stress to which an adopted child is exposed stems from neurotic attitudes on the part of adopting parents, particularly in dealing with his attempts to assert his independence and his ambivalent reactions towards them. Large differences of intelligence between the child and his parents occasionally cause problems, although adoption societies try to avoid this by suitable placing of children.

STEP-CHILDREN

Step-children encounter special difficulties. When the stepmother is insecure and uncertain of her husband's affection, she may be unable to cope with her aggressive feelings for a child, the more so if she has none of her own.

On the other side of the coin, a step-child may feel guilty and responsible for marital discords that develop. Parental quarrels over him lead to deterioration in his standards of behaviour.

CHILDREN IN HOSPITAL—REGRESSION

Any change in family stability makes some children, particularly those before five or six years old, insecure and anxious. A commonplace event such as moving house, father having to go away on a business trip, or the arrival of a new child, may cause anxiety. This may result in *regressive behaviour*. A child who has been previously dry wets the bed, speech may deteriorate, he may cling to his mother and refuse to let her out of his sight, or generally become babyish in his behaviour. This is known as *regression*. Understanding parents see the cause of this and try to be tolerant and more openly affectionate than usual. But over-strict parents may punish this behaviour as being due to naughtiness, thereby increasing the child's insecurity and anxiety.

Separation from his mother is particularly upsetting to a young child. Mother going into hospital is not so bad if the child can remain home with the rest of the family, although her return sometimes results in some degree of regression. More disturbing to the child is his own admission to hospital, although this is now likely to be much less difficult for him than in former times, because doctors and nurses are now beginning to understand the problem. Parents can now visit their children daily in nearly every hospital, and in many hospitals there are no rigid rules or times concerning visiting. Only in fever hospitals and long-stay orthopaedic hospitals, often situated some way from the child's home, are serious psychological difficulties likely to occur.

In the past nurses were sometimes more concerned with the organization of their wards than with the mental welfare of the children. The children were expected to be quiet; the uproar that occurs when parents leave the ward encouraged the idea that visiting 'upset' the child. In fact, the child who screams when his parents leave is reacting in a healthy way to separation. The child who lies quietly in his cot, unresponsive to what is going on round him, is easier to handle but may well be seriously disturbed emotionally.

The acute distress that occurs when a child is separated and brought into hospital has been well recorded in the Robertson's films. At first the child protests loudly, shaking his cot and crying for his mother (period of protest). After a day or so he shows signs of despair and grows silent, although he probably remains preoccupied with the memory of his absent mother. Finally he reaches a stage of detachment, when he appears to be distressed and to lose interest in his parents. Even when his parents do reappear he may pay them little or no attention, and even fail to show recognition of them. When a child returns home after not having seen his mother for several weeks, he is likely to remain detached for some time. Then he begins to show intensely ambivalent feelings, clinging to his mother, demanding all her attention and reacting violently and angrily if she leaves him, even for a few seconds. If the period of separation has lasted for more than six months, and particularly if during this time the child has not received special attention from nurses or visitors, this stage detachment may remain indefinitely and his affections be permanently blunted. Of course, much individual variation in children's reactions exists, but this is typical of children between the ages of six months and four years. Below six months distress is not shown, and it diminishes after four years.

Interesting studies have been carried out on the effect of separation of infant Rhesus monkeys from their mothers. The important factor in the infant's reaction seems to be not so much his separation from his mother as the subsequent disturbance in the mother–infant interaction. When this is not disrupted and particularly when the mother is not upset, there are few ill effects.

How a child will react when he is admitted to hospital depends upon several factors:

1. *Age*. The younger the child, particularly if he is less than two years old, the more likely he is to be upset. After two years it becomes progressively easier to tell him what is going to happen to him and thus to reduce his anxiety. Some hospitals encourage the mother of very young children to come into hospital with the child, but this is not always possible, either for the hospital or the mother. However, the presence of a sibling or of some familiar person will frequently reduce a child's distress.

2. *Family relationships*. A child from a secure, happy home will be less upset than one from an unhappy or broken home. Over-anxious parents are liable to have anxious children and to convey their own anxiety about the admission to the child.

3. *Type of care provided in hospital*. The child's distress can be considerably reduced by the provision of toys, by the reaction of the nurses to him, and how often parents, siblings or friends are able to visit him.

Nurses become temporary mothers to the child. It is usual for each child to have his own special nurse. A screaming child needs to be picked up, not scolded, and the over-quiet two-year-old should not be left alone, but should be given as much attention as possible. This sometimes calls for considerable understanding on the part of the nurse, for the child may not respond emotionally to her at first. Sometimes a nurse may become too attached to a child and feel jealous and resentful towards his mother. But this is exceptional. Most nurses enjoy nursing children and get on well with the parents.

There is little doubt that such separation can have a disturbing effect

51

on a child. On the other hand some children benefit from coming into hospital. An only child, for instance, gains from making friends and learning to play with other children. A deprived child discovers the affection and security that he previously lacked. An over-protected and anxious child may throw off his fears and learn to be more independent.

It is not always remembered that illness, particularly chronic forms such as diabetes or nephritis, cause anxiety and guilt in younger children and make them wonder why they have been singled out for punishment. Children may react to illness by rebelling and becoming unco-operative. Unsympathetic attitudes on the part of nurses and doctors only serve to increase the difficulties. Older children should be encouraged to talk about their fears, the unpleasantness of injections, the general problems of being ill and of being admitted to hospital. Facilities for play or schoolwork are important therapeutically, particularly when long-term hospitalization is involved.

After returning home, and depending to a large extent on how long he has been in hospital, how much he saw of his parents, his age, and how secure his background is, the child may regress in his behaviour and become demanding and difficult. Nurses can help in the child's readjustment by explaining to parents that such behaviour is only a temporary reaction to the insecurity and anxiety he felt in hospital.

HANDICAPPED CHILDREN

Special problems of development arise with handicapped children. They may spend long periods in hospital or be forced to lead restricted lives at home. Any aspect of the child's development may be delayed or distorted in consequence. Unless efforts are made to correct this and help the child to compensate for his deficiencies a vicious circle may arise, leading to still further developmental disturbances.

SCHOOL AGE

A child develops rapidly when he begins to go to school. He admires his teacher and tries to imitate him. He makes friends, learns to give and take, and adopts new ideas and ways of behaviour. He develops a moral sense of right and wrong; he now does this, or does not do that, because that is how those people he respects would behave. At this time the child may have two quite different standards of behaviour: one for school, and one for home. Parents may be astonished to learn their son is a model child at school, tidy and helpful in the classroom and good-natured in play, while at home he is untidy and rude. Sometimes the reverse occurs and the model child may become a destructive devil when he goes to school.

Immature parents may feel jealous of the teacher's influence and try to lower his esteem in the child's eye. This may upset the child. He may feel he must choose between the parents and teacher. He may reject both to become over-dependent or hostile to one or the other. But usually he achieves some sort of compromise! He becomes reasoning and more reasonable. He learns to control his impulses and to behave in ways that are acceptable to society. Theoretically a teacher should be able to retain a more objective view of the child than the parents. But if he is a neurotic personality himself he may be unable to deal fairly with pupils who arouse his anger or anxiety. He may come under pressure from his colleagues or from parents to adopt a more authoritarian and punitive attitude towards his pupils.

By the age of seven or eight most children are reasonably well behaved. From now until just before puberty intellectual growth predominates. *Egocentric thought* gives way to *conceptual and abstract thought*. The child relates objects and ideas to one another in an increasingly complex way. He learns quickly and is constantly searching for fresh stimulation. If he is denied stimulation and is badly taught he may become bored. If he is forced to learn, or if too high a standard for his mental age is demanded. he may rebel against all forms of learning.

PUBERTY (THE STATE OF BECOMING CAPABLE OF SEXUAL REPRODUCTION)

This steady, peaceful development may erupt just before or at puberty. This is a time when widespread psychological and physical changes are occurring. Boys' voices break; girls' breasts begin to develop; hair grows in axillae and pubic areas, and menstruation starts. These changes occur as a result of hormones secreted by the endocrine glands, which help to bring about the physical changes of puberty. These changes in the internal environment also cause psychological changes. Instinctive energies and fantasies, previously well controlled, now make themselves increasingly felt. At first, before the sexual changes of puberty have properly begun, this can lead to aggressive, destructive behaviour.

Boys more than girls may behave in a brutal or cruel manner. Acts of cruelty to animals or to other children may occur. Unruly conduct, destructiveness for its own sake, dirtiness, come and go. Some children, particularly those of obsessive personality, repress their aggressive feelings. As a defence the reverse type of behaviour then occurs. Such children become scrupulously tidy and over-concerned with cleanliness, and need to do good and earn the approval of others. Rituals and compulsive behaviour, designed to ward off evil, sometimes develop. Some children become intensely religious.

Aggressive feelings gradually become tempered by and give way to sexual feelings and behaviour. Today in our society there is a relatively long delay between the time when biological adulthood is reached and independence and sexual freedom are obtained, which creates psychological difficulties. Both sexes increasingly wish to be independent and free from parental ties and restrictions. This often leads to conflict with parents and sometimes to open rejection of parental standards. But underneath the rebellion the adolescent still needs to feel loved and wanted by his parents. If his parents react to his strivings for independence by withdrawing their affection he will become very anxious. Such anxiety will increase his unruly behaviour and a vicious circle may arise.

In place of parents, the adolescent needs to admire some over-valued figure, such as a teacher or film-star. Boys join gangs, which allows them to give vent to their impulses with a sense of security. Frank anti-social behaviour, such as housebreaking or violence, may occur if parental authority has been violently rejected.

Adolescent gangs flourish, particularly in disorganized neighbourhoods, where to some extent they represent attempts to create order out of social chaos. Stealing often occurs as a group activity, members vying to outdare each other. Most adolescents involved in such group behaviour are psychiatrically normal, but at any time the group may come under the influence of one or more seriously disturbed adolescent. Serious antisocial activity and acts of cruelty can then occur.

Contradictory behaviour is characteristic. Idealistic thoughts are mixed with selfishness, intolerance with extreme sensitivity. Both sexes are moody, unpredictable, impulsive and egoistical. Their dogmatic views cover their deep feelings of insecurity. Intelligence reaches its peak of development at sixteen, but experience and therefore wisdom are slight.

Most girls know about *menstruation* at an early age. The average age for menstruation to begin is thirteen, but it can be as early as nine or as late as sixteen. Both early and late menstruation may lead to anxiety and to a fear of being abnormal. Menstruation itself may cause anxiety if fears have been implanted in earlier childhood. The girl may conceal the fact that she has started to menstruate, or make a fuss whenever it occurs. She may feel ashamed and disgusted with her body and starve herself as a means of suppressing and therefore controlling sexual and aggressive feelings. Such behaviour will occasionally progress to *anorexia nervosa* (see p. 125).

Nowadays it is often a matter of prestige that an adolescent should have a partner. Many adolescents, particularly girls, need to fall in love repeatedly before they are ready for marriage. At first this is usually with someone 'safe' and unobtainable; later with someone less remote but still unobtainable, such as the father of a friend. 'Obtainable' men attracted to her are devalued and rejected. Women tend to have a more idealistic fantasy life than males. Although masturbation probably occurs in at least 50 per cent of females, it is not used to relieve sexual tension as commonly as adolescent males. Most males masturbate. Sometimes this sets up guilty feelings, which merely serve to increase sexual tension, and may sometimes result in compulsive masturbation. Both boys and girls may try to suppress their sexual feelings and thoughts by developing intellectual interests by becoming aesthetic or religious, or by other means. Yet others go to the opposite extreme and become vulgar and coarse; the open expression of sexual fears makes them seem less fearful. Most boys feel anxious and uncertain about girls, and *homosexuality* offers a way of escaping their fears. For most adolescents homosexuality is transitory.

Promiscuity, particularly in girls, is more likely to reflect neurotic conflicts and the rejection of parental standards than abnormal sexual urges.

It is virtually impossible to assess the incidence of adolescent psychiatric disorders. Among university students (who probably have a higher rate of breakdown), with access to a Student Health Service, between 1 and 2 per cent develop a serious psychotic illness at some time during their undergraduate life, a further 10–20 per cent have 'neurotic breakdowns', and about the same number experience minor transitory disturbances related to sexual problems, pre-examination nerves, illicit drug taking, and so on.

ADULTHOOD

As the adolescent becomes more self-sufficient and independent so his relationship with his parents improves. He goes to work, enlarges his circles of acquaintances, joins groups and societies, takes on responsibilities, marries and has children of his own.

WORK AND PLAY

A child's play is at first entirely concerned with fantasy, unconcerned with solving problems in the real world. Play gradually changes as the child becomes sociable and relates to his peers, as his intellectual powers widen, and he increasingly co-operates with others. Play gradually merges into work. Work is always directed to a specific end, and should be rational and consciously understood. To work without understanding or aim is frustrating and unsatisfying. In such a situation a man's mental health is often only preserved by his fantasy; the alternative is to direct his interest and energies into outside activities.

Work is an essential part of a man's life, not only for material reasons but psychologically. To work is to be accepted by society and to feel 'useful'. To be unemployed (or even retired) is to feel cut off from society, despised and disregarded. The type of work undertaken depends on intelligence, aptitude, personality and opportunity. Some people of both sexes follow in their parent's footsteps, wishing to emulate or outdo them, others take up entirely different work. Some nurses have felt determined to take up nursing for as long as they can remember. Fantasies, expressed initially in play, often play an important part, particularly in the professions.

The contrast between fantasy and reality may result in psychological difficulties at first. But sooner or later the fantasy and 'the realities of work' will intermingle and produce interest, drive and deep satisfaction.

Girls show maternal feelings from an early age and nursing is a good means of expressing this. Nursing is particularly satisfying work, for not only is it highly regarded by society, but there is pride and a sense of achievement in the work. However, the work is far from easy and it is associated with a good deal of anxiety.

At the lowest level a man works solely to earn money or whatever commodity is necessary for him and his family to exist. Such a man is not able to utilize his fantasies in his work. He will take little pride or interest in his work. He will feel no sense of loyalty or of belonging. There are many reasons for unsatisfactory working conditions, including bad management and lack of communication between management and workers. Boredom and industrial fatigue grow and output falls. A good management instils loyalties in its workers, feeds them with information, makes them feel their job is valuable and that they are necessary. A bored man is a frustrated man, unable to express his feelings satisfactorily.

Accidents reflect not only physical conditions at work but also psychological and social factors. Many accidents occur because of anger, frustration or disappointment. Studies have shown that about 80 per cent of industrial accidents occur only in a small group of workers, comprising about 20 per cent of the total. These people are looked upon as *accident prone*; they tend to be tense, impulsive people who try to relieve their tension by physical activity.

MALE AND FEMALE DIFFERENCES

The greater part of the differences in temperament and behaviour between men and women arises from differences of upbringing. Yet there are constitutional differences present at or shortly after birth. Females sleep longer and are less irritable. There is therefore, perhaps, a tendency for mothers to pick up and hold boys more often than girls. Males tend to be heavier and taller and are physically stronger from the start, although paradoxically females are tougher and survive better. Girls sit up, crawl, walk, and learn to talk earlier than boys. They retain their superiority in verbal skills until puberty. Females are more responsive to auditory stimuli, boys have greater visual acuity and show more interest in visual patterns. This means that from birth the same stimulus will have a somewhat different significance for each sex. Females are more sensitive to pain and touch and more responsive to sweet tastes. Their sense of smell is better developed, particularly after puberty. Boys are more aggressive and competitive in common with most other mammalian species. Girls are more friendly, sympathetic, and protective towards younger children from an early age.

No one description of what constitutes characteristic male or female behaviour is likely to be universally acceptable. A woman from another culture—Indian, Chinese, Egyptian, Italian—is expected to behave very differently from an Englishwoman. But the very word Englishwoman today is misleading, for there are large differences of behaviour between social classes. A working class woman tends to see herself as dominated by the male, her main function being to look after him and raise his children. The upper class woman is more likely to demand equality with the male. The Victorian female, certainly among the middle classes, was looked upon as the devoted custodian of her family or, if unmarried, of her aged parents; the 'angel in the house', gentle, kind, understanding, and self-sacrificing. The Victorian male was looked upon as a hardworking, reliable if stern husband and father, but also sexually demanding and not able to control his appetites in the way females could. Our values and beliefs have profoundly changed over the last century and inevitably our concepts of masculinity and femininity.

SEXUAL DEVELOPMENT

It was Freud who publicized the idea of infantile sexuality. It is important to understand what is meant by the term and to distinguish it from adult or genital sexuality. Children derive considerable pleasure from stimulating their bodies, including their genitalia, from an early age, and orgasmic-like reactions can be observed in young children. Erection of the penis may occur shortly after birth, and is not a foretaste of superhuman virility but a reflex response to a full rectum. Infants begin to play with their genitals from around 5 months onwards, boys more so than girls. Ejaculation can only occur however after puberty is reached.

Sex play and self-stimulation during early childhood is not only pleasurable but comforting to the child. From three or four years onwards, sexual activities involving other children or adults are common, reflecting curiosity, pleasure and excitement. Genital exploration and display is a common feature of childhood with both sexes. Oral sex is common, but attempts at actual genital intercourse are probably uncommon in our society.

Freud pointed out the existence of erotogenic zones of the body, stimulation of which gave particular pleasure: the mouth, anus, and genital organs. He thought that in the normal process of maturation these erotogenic zones lost their sensual qualities, and sexual pleasure eventually became confined to the genital areas. He described childhood sexuality as 'polymorphus perverse', meaning that all erotic potentialities were explored by the child through his own body or through the bodies of others, directly or at a distance, by touching and watching. It is man's prolonged childhood which creates the complexities of adult sexuality. But in fact childhood sexuality is not repressed. Far from it, genital sexual satisfaction should follow on from 'polymorphus perverse' foreplay. Without that childlike love play which precedes intercourse, sexuality is dull and unsatisfying.

By the age of seven about 10 per cent of boys masturbate quite frequently and this proportion rises steadily, with a rapid increase just before and after puberty. Girls follow boys in this pattern, but with a lower incidence. The majority of pre-adolescent and young pubescent girls suppress their sexual feelings or project them on to some unattainable celebrity. At puberty sexual drives direct the adolescent towards his sexual object, which may or may not be attainable, and push sexual fantasies into consciousness. It is now that fears arise, often connected with underlying fantasies, and the adolescent becomes anxious, fearing that he will never be able to lead a normal sexual life. This will force him increasingly into more fantasy.

Sexual excitement brings about widespread physiological changes. The erection of penis and clitoris is the result of their engorgement with blood. The penis can expand to two or three times its resting size and double its width. The clitoris becomes erect and swollen to twice its normal size, together with the lips around the entrance of the vagina. Breasts and nipples, ear lobes, lips, nose, anus, are all similarly engorged and sexually responsive. The pulse and blood pressure rise, reaching a sudden peak at orgasm. Respiration increases and becomes deeper and gasping at orgasm. Salivary secretion increases and may be profuse. As orgasm approaches perception alters, sensation is diminished and narrowed and may be momentarily lost during orgasm. Quite severe injuries, which would normally cause considerable pain, may go unfelt until after orgasm. The face becomes contorted as the facial muscles tense up, the mouth opens and gasps for air. Eyes are either shut or stare blankly into the distance. At orgasm tension reaches a peak and is then suddenly released in a series of convulsions and muscular spasms, which may be localized or affect the whole body, and last anything up to several minutes. In some people these spasms may be extremely painful. Ejaculation usually accompanies a man's orgasm but is not an essential part of it.

Male and female both take about the same time to reach orgasm by masturbation. Provided the female is already sexually aroused when intercourse begins she can usually reach orgasm as quickly as the male. But in practice most people like to prolong their intercourse.

MARRIAGE

Sooner or later the question of marriage will arise. The rate of illegitimate births in Britain has risen sharply over the past 15 years, but no one doubts that our society is still based upon the family. Russia attempted to abolish the family after the 1917 Revolution but the scheme met with failure. And even the Kibbutz system in Israel, in which the children are brought up collectively, still preserves the basis of family life; children join their parents for part of each day.

Marriage satisfies both biological and psychological needs. Women, because they mature earlier, tend to marry younger. They differ from men in that the biological need for conception and motherhood is perhaps present from an early age. This may show itself in an open desire to have babies, or alternatively in loud denials of any such wish. It is often important for a woman to invest her future husband with desirable and exaggerated qualities. This helps her to separate from her family and to accept her role as a wife. Her husband also responds to the idea of being a superman. His self-esteem and confidence increase, together with a new sense of responsibility. After marriage, of course, both will become more realistic towards one another, and both will have to make adjustments in their outlook and behaviour in order for the relationship to develop.

Teenage marriages are increasing. The availability of contraceptive pills, by removing the risk of pregnancy, ensures that a high proportion of teenagers of both sexes now have sexual relationships. Women tend to form more stable relationships than men and there is little doubt that a satisfying sexual relationship produces a strong 'bonding' effect. Some teenagers are mature individuals, emotionally ready for marriage. But many are emotionally unstable and may marry simply in order to escape from their parents, to gain security, and so on. They may invest their partners with such unrealistic qualities that they may be unable to deal with the realities of marriage.

The seriousness with which society regards marriage is exemplified in the marriage ceremony; this not only sets the approval of society on the two people living together, it also highlights the fact that society accepts them as adults and expects them to behave responsibly.

SEXUAL INTERCOURSE

Sexual intercourse that is satisfying to both partners is an essential part of a happy marriage. Male potency and female receptivity depend upon a number of factors, perhaps the most important being the sexual fantasies of each partner and the way in which these relate or correspond to the attitudes and feelings of one for the other. Some men do not derive much pleasure from intercourse with their wives and regard it more as a duty, only being able to enjoy intercourse with a mistress or a prostitute, or preferring masturbation. This pattern of behaviour is relatively uncommon in women. Men do not always realize that an adequate period of love-making must precede coitus if their wives are to experience orgasm. Anxiety in either partner may have unfortunate results. Men are liable to become impotent and this is not uncommon on the first night of a honeymoon. Women are more likely to experience pain (*dyspareunia*). In either case, a vicious circle may perpetuate this situation.

However, the majority of married people gradually learn to adjust to one another and sooner or later pregnancy will probably occur.

59

PSYCHOLOGY AND PSYCHIATRY FOR NURSES

Pregnancy brings about both physiological and psychological changes, each tending to affect and be affected by the other. Many women tend to become more passive and 'cowlike', due perhaps to the *progesterone* produced by the developing *placenta*.

The first three months are often the most difficult. Not only has the woman to come to terms with, and accept her pregnancy; she may also have to cope with nausea and sickness, and overcome feelings of exhaustion and depression. The early nausea and tiredness are probably due to one or more of the physiological changes of pregnancy. Usually these symptoms disappear by the fourth month, but occasionally vomiting increases and continues throughout most of the pregnancy. Although some cases may be primarily psychological in origin, in many instances psychiatric disturbances are the result rather than the cause of the vomiting.

Mood changes often occur in women at certain times in pregnancy. The extent of these changes depends to some extent on the personality of the woman. Women with *obsessive personalities* usually feel on top of the world when they are pregnant. Women with *hysterical* personalities are often depressed and emotionally unstable throughout their pregnancies.

Depression is particularly liable to occur in the first three months, but usually disappears by the fourth month. It may recur in the last weeks of pregnancy. Emotional instability and irritability are common. Anxiety may come and go. It may express itself as a fear that the baby will be born deformed or dead, that childbirth will kill her, or that her husband will leave her. Much of the anxiety can be dealt with by reassurance and explanation given in antenatal classes.

During pregnancy appetites, like moods, fluctuate. There are sudden cravings for unusual foods, or foods previously avoided or disliked. And food normally enjoyed may now be avoided. Compulsive over-eating sometimes occurs, particularly in tense, worried women, leading to large and undesirable weight gains.

Sexual desire often fluctuates. Some women lose all feelings from the time they conceive; others have increased desire, though this usually starts to diminish from mid-pregnancy onwards. Unless husband and wife appreciate that these changes are to be expected, difficulties may arise.

Difficulties may also occur as a result of the woman becoming more passive and wanting to be given love and affection. The husband may resent this and refuse to pander to his wife's whims. The resentment may be increased by his wife's depression or irritability. Often a straightforward talk by a nurse, with both together, will break a vicious circle.

Very few women can 'imagine' the foetus or even appreciate fully that they are pregnant until they begin to feel movements. Feelings for a child then gradually develop and it becomes real to them, but the mental image of the child may remain rather featureless until after the delivery. Sometimes, however, vivid dreams of the baby may occur both by day and by night. At birth the mother may feel intense emotion when she is handed the baby. But it is also not uncommon, particularly when labour has been long and distressing, for a mother to feel no emotion whatever at the sight of her child. Maternal feeling will then appear some time later. In most instances a satisfactory mother–child relationship will develop within the first week, particularly when breast-feeding begins.

As we have already implied, pregnancy makes demands on the husband. He has to understand his wife's emotional lability and give her support and affection. He has to accept the child and to adapt himself to the fact that his wife is also now a mother. He may have to juggle with jealousy towards the child and resentment over his wife not giving him so much of her time as before. Some husbands experience sympathetically some of their wives' symptoms during pregnancy or childbirth. This is known as the *Couvarde syndrome*.

DELIVERY AND THE PUERPERIUM

Childbirth is sometimes looked upon as rather a frightening process. Antenatal classes, talks, relaxation, and exercises have not entirely dispelled this fear, although it is probably very much less now than it was twenty or thirty years ago.

Today women are encouraged to have their first babies in hospital. Sometimes conditions in the labour ward are far from satisfactory. Women may be left alone in labour for several hours, frightened and in pain. Labour may be prolonged by the woman's own anxiety. Overworked midwives may become impatient and tell the woman to hurry up or to stop behaving like a baby. Resentment and guilt builds up. An exhausted, demoralized, miserable woman may have little emotional feeling for her child when at last he is born. Husbands are now sometimes encouraged to be with their wives during labour or part of it. But not all husbands and wives take kindly to this. Epidural techniques of delivery have made a tremendous difference to some women, allowing them to experience childbirth in full consciousness without pain and misery.

As soon as the child is born, he is usually handed to his mother. Most women experience a surge of pleasure and satisfaction at this moment. This experience is lessened if the mother has been bullied or treated unsympathetically during her labour, or if she has been too heavily sedated or anaesthetized. Apart from the value of this experience in stimulating maternal feelings, many women become very anxious if they do not see the child, fearing that he is deformed or dead.

Breast-feeding is usually encouraged in hospital, although there is disagreement as to how far women should be persuaded to do it. Some women feel disgusted and embarrassed by breast-feeding and will become anxious and upset if they are forced to conform. Modern artificial foods are probably as good nutritionally as breast milk, and an infant certainly cannot distinguish a bottle from a breast in his first weeks of life. But there is little doubt that many mothers experience increased maternal feelings

61

when they breast-feed, and this may result in the breast-fed infant being fondled more than the bottle-fed one. Recent work has suggested that it is the amount of handling that a child receives rather than the way he is fed that influences his early development.

Many women feel depressed during the first week after the delivery. They cry for trivial reasons, feel that they will never be able to cope alone with the child or worry because they think they do not feel the appropriate love for the baby. Sympathy and encouragement will usually help mothers and their husbands over this sometimes difficult phase.

Some mothers love their children to be totally dependent upon them and these women are often model mothers for young babies. Sometimes a woman loses interest as her children become independent. Women of strongly obsessional personality may have difficulty in coping with their children when they are two or three, unable to relax the feeling that they must be completely in control of the relationship and what is going on. Another woman may dislike the helpless state of a young baby, and only begin to enjoy her children later when she feels that they have a real and separate existence apart from her.

THE UNMARRIED MOTHER AND PREGNANCY

In addition to all the difficulties discussed above, the unmarried woman often lacks security and has to fend for herself during pregnancy, It is frequently said that most unmarried mothers are emotionally disturbed and have received little affection in their childhood. The pregnancy is thought to satisfy the girl's longing for someone to love, and who will love her. At the same time, by her behaviour she gets her own back on her parents. It is doubtful if this applies to more than a small proportion of unmarried mothers. Extra-marital intercourse is widespread today. Many factors probably help to determine whether a girl becomes pregnant, and if she does so whether she has an abortion, keeps her child or has him adopted.

THE ABORTION ACT

The Abortion Act of 1967 allows pregnancy to be terminated provided two registered practitioners agree that (a) the life of the woman, or her physical or mental health, or the mental health of any existing children in the family would be threatened if the pregnancy continued; or (b) there is a risk that the child will be born suffering from serious physical or mental abnormalities. In 1971 in England and Wales there were 126 777 legal terminations. (30 000 of these were foreign women from Europe). Just over half the English women terminated were single, and most were aged 24 or less. Most of the married women terminated had already had two or more children and were over 30. The role of the psychiatrist in deciding whether or not termination should occur has altered greatly over the past five years. His main task now is not to say whether a woman should have a termination, but to advise the obstetrician whether or not a patient is likely to develop psychological sequelae following termination. This is never an easy matter, but in general termination seems to have few adverse psychiatric effects in previously stable women with good reason for wanting termination, whether married or single. On the other hand neurotic, inadequate women are liable to feel considerable guilt after termination, and for years afterwards may centre their difficulties around this 'loss'. Of women refused termination, at least 1 in 4 achieve it by 'other means'. There is evidence from Sweden that children born after their mothers have been refused a therapeutic abortion are more likely to develop psychiatric and educational disabilities than other children.

WORKING WIVES

Once the children go to school, either nursery school or primary school, many mothers feel a need to go out to work. They may become depressed or discontented if they have only their homes to look after. They need the stimulation and the companionship of others. Some husbands object to their wives working, feeling that their own status is thereby diminished; and they may resent their wives having independence and a life in which they play no part. Such men usually have insecure and immature personalities. There is reason to think that women who want to go out to work and do so are psychologically healthier as a result, and able to give more to their children.

DIVORCE AND SEPARATION

These invariably affect the children, although not necessarily adversely. The earlier the breakup occurs in a child's life, the greater the effect on his mental development. But separation may be preferable if there are continual scenes between parents, although much depends on the circumstances of the children after separation. It is better to send a child to a good institution, or for the child to be brought up by one parent, than for him to continue living in a home torn by quarrelling and strife. A child from such a hostile environment is likely to become antisocial and aggressive in behaviour. It is the quarrelling and unhappiness that may precede divorce that damages a child's development.

THE SINGLE ADULT

Until comparatively recently there was a great excess of women over men. Spinsterdom was, therefore, inevitable for many women. Men, on the other hand, could mostly choose whether or not to marry.

63

Men and women who choose to remain single throughout their lives are often inhibited, rather unbending personalities, afraid to form a deep emotional relationship with the opposite sex. They make a niche for themselves in life, concentrate on their work or hobbies, and unless they are unsettled by some unforeseen event, such as a serious illness, they remain reasonably, if narrowly, adjusted.

But the single women whose state has been imposed upon her by circumstances may have difficulty in maintaining a satisfactory adjustment. Many *sublimate* their sexual feelings in their work and perform an invaluable role in the community, for example, as teachers or nurses. Some tend inevitably to be immature and form immature relationships. They often make devoted friends but may ultimately become so possessive and demanding that the relationship disintegrates.

The single woman may derive intense satisfaction from her work but sometimes as she approaches the age of forty sexual feelings again begin to be felt. A chance affair may make her feelings uncontrollable. She may resort to *masturbation* as a means of relieving tension. Guilt and anxiety usually follow. At this stage she may tell a doctor or nurse of her anxieties. Simple reassurance will often do a great deal of good and enable her to deal with her impulses. Isolation is particularly dangerous at this time and the single women should be encouraged to join a club or social group.

MIDDLE AGE

Middle age is often a time of contentment and stability for a man, provided he is secure in his work and home. But it is also potentially a dangerous time. He may feel that his ambitions will never be achieved and that he is a failure. He may unexpectedly lose his job for reasons beyond his control and be unable to find a comparable position. Financial problems cause mounting anxiety. He may become seriously depressed and feel that he cannot carry on living.

A women may also encounter these problems but other factors also arise. She must adjust to the physiological changes that occur at the *menopause*. Control over emotions and impulses may be upset. She may feel that the menopause represents the end of her life as a woman and that she will no longer be attractive. Difficulties may be increased for the married woman when her children grow up and leave home. For some mothers the idea of their children leaving home or becoming engaged to marry is extremely difficult to accept. A daughter's sexual behaviour usually has a far more profound effect on her mother than a son's. The mother's repressed sexual conflicts, resentments towards her spouse, regrets at her own lost opportunities, may suddenly erupt and create a family crisis. Loss of parents or close friends may be particularly upsetting to those who are unmarried.

Of course, many women go through the menopause without any

symptoms. This is most likely to happen when the woman is leading a full and satisfying life, and is not completely dependent upon her family.

Sexual interest and activity will depend largely on the personalities. Some men and women slowly lose interest and potency from middle age onwards. Others react to middle age by increased sexual activity. The cessation of menstruation need have little effect on a woman's sexual responses. In fact some women are able to respond sexually much more when their fear of pregnancy is gone. Women who have never accepted or enjoyed their sexual role may use the menopause to bring their sexual life to a close. This frequently leads to marital disturbances and sometimes results in husbands looking elsewhere for their sexual satisfaction.

Many women are now on long-term oestrogen substitution therapy, which seems to have many advantages, both physically and psychologically.

There is no equivalent male menopause. Testosterone levels continue undiminished until old age, although it seems likely that the 'target organs or centres', particularly in the hypothalamus, become less sensitive to the hormones. There is no reason why people of both sexes should not continue sexual activity, relatively undiminished, until old age.

OLD AGE

Biological ageing occurs in everyone, but its effects vary widely from one person to another. Some families start to age when relatively young, while others are still young and adaptable at eighty years old.

Retirement may be felt as a serious loss by a man, especially if he has no outside interests to turn to. He may become bitterly aware of his lost status and look upon himself as a 'has been'. In many societies the old are respected. In our society they are all too often ignored or despised by those who are young and vigorous.

No one fully understands what happens with ageing, but there is a progressive decrease in energy and strength and ability to stand up to stress of all kinds. Physiological adaptation is impaired. A relatively mild infection or injury is enough to kill an old person. Widespread bodily changes occur. The cardiovascular system is less efficient and the blood supply to the brain may be seriously diminished. Brain cells die. Sensation, including vision and hearing, may decrease. At first these defects are covered by substitutions, but eventually disorganization occurs, with the threat of a breakdown.

Certain mental changes characterizing ageing:

1. Old people become self-centred, introspective and egocentric, and are often over-sensitive and quick to take offence.

2. They become increasingly unadaptable in their outlook and behaviour. Anything new or strange is rejected at once and compared unfavourably with the past. New skills cannot be learnt.

3. Memory for recent events fails, but incidents of long ago are

remembered vividly. As a result old people may come to live increasingly in the past, particularly if they lead isolated lives and lack the stimulation provided by young and more active people.

4. Depression, anxiety and a sense of isolation are common. There is increasing preoccupation with bodily functions (*hypochondriasis*) partly because of the anxiety aroused by the death of friends or relatives, and partly because of the bodily changes which occur with ageing. Worry about bowels is particularly common.

5. The usual sleep rhythm may be reversed and the old person will get up at night. In the dark he may become disorientated and confused.

6. Control over appetite and impulses may diminish. Eating habits may become dirty and coarse. There may be abnormal sexual behaviour, offences against children or *exhibitionism*. Aggressive outbursts, greed and a loss of moral sense are distressing to the relatives.

Between 1951 and 1968 the pensionable population rose by 2 million to 8.5 million and the number of people over 75 increased by 700 000 to 2.5 million. The percentage of old people, particularly in the group 75 and over, will continue to increase until about the end of the century. Women greatly outnumber men. About 2 per cent of the elderly are in residential care, but many more are being cared for by devoted relatives. It has been suggested that about 10 per cent of the elderly need residential care, but this would require an enormous expansion of resources.

GRIEF AND MOURNING

In every human society the death of someone who is loved causes grief. Mourning follows. Although the outward signs of mourning may vary with nationality and religion, there is a characteristic sequence of psychological events.

At first the individual may refuse to accept the idea of death. He may throw himself on the body and try to revive it. This may be followed by a sense of numbness. He may sit or walk about in a daze for some time. In extreme cases the initial denial of death may persist. He may continue to speak of the dead person as though he were still alive. Visual hallucinations are not at all uncommon; a face or the complete person may be seen by the griever. Auditory hallucinations are rare. The majority of these hallucinations occur when dropping off to sleep or waking up. Vivid dreams of the dead person are also very common.

But gradually reality returns and he comes to accept the death. He now has an acute sense of loss. Painful memories fill his mind. He weeps, often in the company of friends or relatives who share his sorrow; this helps him to express his feelings appropriately, a necessary process if his grief is to be fully resolved.

He continues to think and speak of the dead person for a variable time. But gradually his feelings become less painful and he comes to interest himself again in other people. He may adopt some of the qualities of the dead person that he particularly admired, or take on some of his responsibilities. Sometimes mourning lasts as long as a year, but eventually it is complete. He can now think realistically and with reasonable detachment about the dead person.

Occasionally grief continues indefinitely. The smallest reference to the dead person causes an emotional outburst. People who react in this way may rebuild their lives around the dead person, even going so far as to preserve the dead person's possessions or rooms exactly as they were in life.

Similar grief reactions, although varying in degree, may occur after any sense of loss. They follow events such as the failure of a marriage, failure at work, or amputation of a limb.

Grief can remain severe for between six and twelve weeks, but then begins to decline. However it may continue for much longer and eventually become so severe as to require admission to hospital. The loss of a spouse is associated with an increased risk of suicide; in the following year the risk is about $2\frac{1}{2}$ times greater than normal. But mortality is also increased among the bereaved from other causes. During the first 4 years of bereavement there is a greatly increased risk, for widowers in particular, of coronary thrombosis and arteriosclerotic heart disease. This risk is particularly high during the first six months following bereavement.

7

CONSCIOUSNESS AND THE UNCONSCIOUS

There are many definitions of consciousness. By the term *consciousness* we mean a person's state of *awareness*. *Awareness* consists of sensations ideas, memories, emotions, and so on. The range of consciousness, or state of awareness, varies from one person to another. A new-born child is conscious of little apart from unsatisfied needs. Consciousness is reduced by alcohol and depressant drugs, by sleep, illness or fatigue. Awareness may be heightened by emotion.

We are never fully conscious of everything that happens around us. Certain things receive full attention, others are totally ignored. Between these two extremes events and objects may be more or less partially noticed. Consciousness therefore can be conveniently pictured as being made up of three concentric circles.

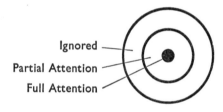

FIGURE 7.1

The term subconscious is used here to include all mental activity outside consciousness at any moment. You may be engrossed in a book when suddenly you remember that you must phone your mother at a certain number. Until that moment the thought and the telephone number were held in the subconscious part of your mind, although readily available.

Many of our mental processes go on subconsciously. You may have a difficult problem to solve or a decision to make. Having thought about it fruitlessly all day you eventually go to bed in despair. Next morning you wake up with the problem solved.

The term *unconscious* is used by us to refer to that part of the mind which contains memories inaccessible to consciousness by ordinary means. An unpleasant event that occurred in the past may be completely

68

'forgotten' (repression). No amount of trying on the part of the person concerned will recall it. But under *hypnosis*, or under the influence of certain drugs, the unconscious memories and feelings may be brought into consciousness. Conversely, during deep hypnosis a subject may be instructed to perform some action after waking. At the same time he is told that he will not remember the instructions. When the time comes he will then automatically carry out the order, although he will have no recollection then or later of having been told to do so. Unconscious material may therefore influence conscious behaviour.

Unconscious memories are also brought to light during *psychoanalysis* by 'free association'. The subject allows his thoughts to wander without conscious direction, and after a time material from the unconscious begins to emerge.

SLEEP

Our understanding of sleeping and dreaming has been greatly increased by the application of the electro-encephalogram to human sleep. Sleep is of two kinds: (1) Rapid eye movement (REM) or paradoxical sleep which takes up to 25 per cent of the night's sleep, and (2) Non-rapid eye movement (NREM) or orthodox sleep, which is subdivided into four stages, the fourth stage producing the slowest waves on the electro-encephalogram.

REM and NREM sleep alternate with each other every 60–90 minutes during normal sleep. REM sleep always follows stage two of NREM. REM sleep is accompanied by eye movements, increased blood flow to the brain, fluctuations of pulse, blood pressure and respiration, and erection of the penis. On waking from REM sleep dreams are clearly remembered and reported. But mental activity occurs at all stages of sleep, and in orthodox sleep has a conscious thoughtlike content. For instance, on waking from orthodox sleep a man will often report that he has been thinking of the day's events.

Patients with coronary insufficiency sometimes develop angina at night. This is most likely to occur during REM sleep and least during stage four of deep sleep. Duodenal ulcer patients frequently waken with pain after two or three hours sleep. They tend to secrete large amounts of gastric juice at night, and it is now known that maximum secretion occurs during REM sleep. Sleepwalking and night terrors are related to deep sleep, which is why they are not remembered. Nightmares, on the other hand, occur during paradoxical sleep. Depressive illness is associated with reduction of stage four of orthodox sleep.

Many drugs upset the normal balance between these two stages of sleep. Barbiturates suppress paradoxical sleep. If they are continued for any length of time tolerance builds up. Stopping the drug results in REM rebound, with insomnia or restless sleep and vivid unpleasant nightmares. It is because of this rebound phenonemon that so many people become habituated to their hypnotic. Indeed it seems likely that REM rebound is intimately related to the addictiveness of any drug: it occurs with amphetamines, alcohol and most hypnotics.

Both kinds of sleep are necessary, and deprivation of either or both can cause perceptual and mood disturbances, and be followed later by rebound. It is now known that the large nocturnal output of growth hormone, which is concerned in the synthesis of ribonucleic acid and protein into the blood, is dependent on orthodox sleep. It may well be that orthodox sleep helps to restore body tissues, while paradoxical sleep is linked with synthetic and restorative functions in the brain.

8

THE PHYSICAL BASIS OF PSYCHOLOGY

So far we have been discussing mental processes and functions. Now we must briefly describe the physical structures upon which these mental processes depend.

NEURONES AND NERVE IMPULSE

Neurones are the structural units of the nervous system. They are made up of a cell body, with protoplasmic outgrowths known as *axons* and

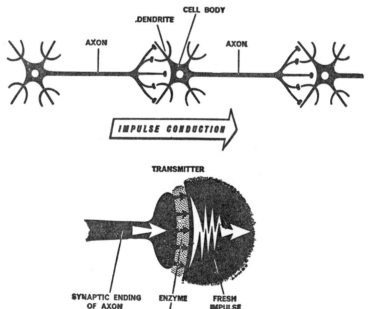

FIGURE 8.1

dendrites. When the cell body is stimulated an electric signal, the *nerve impulse*, is transmitted along the axon. The axon ends at a *synaptic junction*, separated by a short gap from dendrites of neighbouring neurones. The nerve impulse does not jump this gap. Its arrival at a synaptic cleft releases a neurotransmitter substance from vesicles in which it is stored at the end of the axon. This diffuses across the synaptic cleft to the neighbouring dendrites. Depending upon its nature, the neurotransmitter may produce excitation, causing a new impulse to be set up in the next neurone, or it will set up a state of inhibition, reducing the excitability of the neurone. The action of the neurotransmitter is shortlived. Most of it is rapidly taken up again into the end of the axon, the rest being destroyed by enzymic activity.

That acetylcholine and noradrenaline are the neurotransmitters in the peripheral nervous system has long been known. Our knowledge of neurotransmitters within the brain itself is much less clear. Noradrenaline, serotonin, dopamine, acetylcholine, have been identified among others. Noradrenaline has been identified in the hypothalamus and midbrain areas and seems to be concerned with mood and reward signalling systems. Serotonin is scattered through the midbrain and perhaps influences mood, perception and sleep. The action of antidepressant drugs is believed to be due to their ability either to prevent the reuptake of a neurotransmitter or to prevent its destruction (see p. 185).

BRAIN

The anatomical pathways and physiological mechanisms of emotion and thought are only just beginning to be understood. Not so long ago the *brain* was thought to be made up of ascending layers with the *cerebral cortex* at the top and in control. It is true that we owe our superiority of intelligence to the development and differentiation of the cerebral cortex But we now realize that there is continual interaction between one part of the brain and another, and that the brain acts as an integrated whole. Not only does the cortex influence subcortical structures, but these in turn affect the cortex.

The cortex can be divided from the point of view of its evolutionary development, into an old *visceral cortex*, and a comparatively new *neocortex*. In lower animals the visceral cortex is concerned with smell and emotional expression. In man the relationship of the visceral cortex to emotional expression has been retained. The neocortex seems to be mainly concerned with intelligence. It is significant that the visceral cortex and subcortical structures of man have not evolved to anything like the same extent as the neocortex. These probably provide the emotional background against which man functions intellectually.

Below the cortex are the *hypothalamus* and the *thalamus*.

The most interesting (in terms of current knowledge) subcortical structures are the hypothalamus, ascending reticular activating system and the limbic system. The ascending reticular system stretches from the bulbar region to the medial thalamus. It is intimately involved in wakefulness, general alertness and attention. Wakefulness demands a constant inflow of sensory stimuli, and this is relayed through the reticular system. Damage or destruction to the ascending reticular system causes sleepiness, inattention and general lack of interest.

The *limbic system* is a complex of structures lying around the intraventricular foramina in the cerebral hemispheres, intimately involved with the temporal lobes. It includes the hippocampus, amygdala, cingulate and dentate gyri. The main connections of the system are with the reticular formation and the frontal lobes.

The limbic system is concerned with emotional experience, expression and behaviour. Removal of both temporal lobes in monkeys, including the amygdala and most of the hippocampus, produces what is known as the Kluver–Bucy syndrome: increased and often perverse sexual activity, over-eating, visual agnosia and lack of fear. Bilateral amygdalectomy alone results in hypersexuality and over-eating. It seems that the amygdala exerts an inhibitory controlling influence within the system. In cats, hypersexuality following amygdalectomy can be abolished by destroying the ventral nuclei of the hypothalamus. Similar operations have been carried out on humans with uncontrollable antisocial sexual perversions, with some degree of success.

Bilateral removal of the hippocampus upsets memory and learning of the type which demands comparison of one stimulus with another. Suppose, for instance, two stimuli separated by a short gap are given to an animal. The animal responds in one way when the stimuli are identical, in another when different, and is rewarded (or not punished) when successful. In order to learn this the animal must be able to retain the memory of the first stimulus and compare it to the second. Hippocampal animals cannot do this. *Korsakov syndrome*, a complication of alcoholism, is associated with damage to the hippocampus.

The hypothalamus, lying in the diencephalon, plays a major role in homeostasis, in controlling the body's internal needs, and in maintaining a fine balance between input and output. Its influence extends over body temperature, food and water balance, sex functions, cardiovascular and gastro-intestinal functions.

The hypothalamus contains large collections of neurones (nuclei) which control and integrate endocrine and autonomic nervous system activities. It exerts a direct influence on posterior pituitary hormones. For instance, antidiuretic hormone is produced in the hypothalamus and travels via nerve trunks to the pituitary to release vasopressin. Anterior pituitary hormones such as growth hormone and gonadotrophins are controlled by hypothalamic substances which travel to the pituitary via the portal blood vessel system. A sensitive feedback system allows a very fine control to be maintained.

There are well-defined 'centres' within the hypothalamus. Thus, stimulation of part of the medial hypothalamus decreases the amount of food eaten. Destruction of this area causes over-eating. Stimulation of the lateral part produces over-eating. Anorexia follows its destruction. In the normal state a balance seems to exist between these two centres. Hypothalamic disturbances are common in psychiatric disorders. In anorexia nervosa for instance, the onset of amenorrhoea is almost certainly due to hypothalamic factors.

The *autonomic nervous system* controls internal organs, such as the heart and bowels and secretory glands which cannot be voluntarily controlled. The system is composed of *sympathetic* and *parasympathetic* divisions. Although these two divisions have opposing actions, they normally co-operate and so produce a delicate regulating system. *Sympathetic activity* dilates the pupil, increases the heart rate, dries the mouth, blanches the skin and brings on a cold sweat, raises blood pressure, inhibits peristalsis and causes muscle sphincters to contract. In addition, the adrenal medulla is stimulated to secrete *adrenaline*. *Adrenaline* not only reinforces sympathetic activity, but releases sugar into the blood from the liver. Erection of the penis depends upon sympathetic activity.

Parasympathetic activity slows the heart, constricts bronchioles, increases the flow of saliva and peristaltic movement, and causes muscle sphincters to relax. Insulin secretion from the pancreas is stimulated, leading to a fall of blood sugar.

The autonomic system prepares the body for fight or flight when danger arises. At such times sympathetic activity predominates. But the autonomic system also serves to maintain homeostasis through its control of respiration, temperature regulation, digestion and excretion, blood distribution and so on. For this purpose the parasympathetic system predominates.

THE PHYSICAL BASIS OF EMOTION

What happens within the brain when we experience fear or anger at the sight of danger?

1. The hypothalamus is alerted from the thalamus and by direct branches from the reticular system. From the hypothalamus there occur *simultaneously*:

(a) An upward discharge of nerve impulses to the old visceral cortex; particularly important is the limbic system. This results in emotional feeling and the need for some kind of action.

(b) A downward discharge through the sympathetic and para-sympathetic centres and the pituitary gland. *This results in appropriate bodily changes.*

2. The neocortex is alerted to the danger through its associations with the limbic lobe and the reticular system. *The action required to meet the situation is rapidly decided and begun.*

In emotional states, such as fear, sympathetic activity predominates. In others, such as grief, parasympathetic activity is more marked. But individual differences are great; sympathetic or parasympathetic activity

THE PHYSICAL BASIS OF PSYCHOLOGY

may always predominate in some people's reactions. One student always has frequency or diarrhoea (parasympathetic effects) before an important exam, another develops sympathetic overactivity with tachycardia, a dry mouth, and inability to keep still.

THE GENERAL ADAPTATION SYNDROME (G.A.S.)

Hans Selye believes that when someone is put under a stress two kinds of reaction occur in the body. The first is a local reaction, which depends on the nature of the stress, such as a burn or a cut. The second is a general reaction of the body, which is always the same no matter what the stress may be. This general reaction he calls the *general adaptation syndrome* (G.A.S.).

He describes three stages in its development. The first stage is the *Alarm reaction*, which is comparatively short. The autonomic nervous system becomes active, *adrenaline* is discharged into the blood stream, and *adrenocorticotrophic hormone* (A.C.T.H.) is secreted by the pituitary gland. This stimulates the adrenal cortex to produce its hormones.

If it survives this stage the body adapts to the stress, and the *stage of resistance* begins. This may last for years, but if the stress continues for long enough eventually the *stage of exhaustion* occurs. Physiological mechanisms begin to fail and symptoms of illness appear. When homeostasis can no longer be maintained death results.

Selye has called those illnesses showing the symptoms of this last stage *diseases of adaptation*. It is questionable as to how far this theory can be applied to mental disease. But analogous stages are apparent in fighting men during battle. Efficiency and alertness increase rapidly to a peak, which is maintained for a variable time. Sooner or later exhaustion occurs, alertness diminishes, and men begin to break down.

PART TWO

PSYCHIATRY

9

MENTAL DISORDERS

HISTORICAL

Mental disorders have existed throughout recorded history. The Greeks and Romans treated their own mentally ill members (but not their slaves) with reasonable tolerance and understanding. With the arrival of Christianity attitudes towards the mentally ill began to change. Mental illness came to be equated with the Devil and his works. This came to a head during the Middle Ages, and for three centuries the mentally ill, particularly female, were persecuted and burnt as witches.

During the 18th century a more humane and enlightened attitude towards the mentally ill began to spread through Europe. People were repelled by the way the insane were treated. At the end of the 18th century the Frenchman Pinel freed patients in the Bicêtre from their chains. In England, William Tuke founded The Retreat at York. He forbade the use of chains and manacles and patients were treated with respect and kindness. This 'moral treatment' of the insane created widespread interest and concern. Eventually an investigation into conditions in madhouses was set up in 1815, which revealed a horrifying state of affairs. But already in 1808 a bill to provide for the better treatment of the insane had been introduced. Amending bills eventually led to the creation of the Lunacy Commission.

Mental hospitals now began to be built throughout the country. These were often very large, with 2000 or more beds, situated well away from the large towns from which they drew their patients. The enlightened views of the early reformers gradually gave way to indifference and apathy among the staff. Patients were herded together in locked wards, often heavily sedated and given little or no opportunity to develop self respect and initiative. They were in a sense social outcasts, segregated from normal people and herded together like animals. By the Lunacy Act of 1890 *only certified* patients could be admitted to a mental hospital, and this remained so until the Act of 1930. This Act allowed mental hospitals to admit patients on a voluntary basis. In 1948 the National Health Service was created and overnight all hospitals, general and mental, were taken over by the State and given equal status and financial help. Morale among the staff of mental hospitals rose and spread to their patients. New forms of management were introduced and efforts made to counteract the deadening effects of institutionalism. Doors were unlocked and the concept of a *therapeutic community* put into practice. Patients were treated as dignified human beings allowed freedom and independence. All this was enormously helped by the introduction in the early 1950s of the phenothiazine group of tranquillizers and, a few years later, the anti-depressants. The 1959 Mental Health Act completed the process of abolishing the statutory distinction between mental and physical illness. From now on any hospital might admit the mentally ill, whether on a compulsory section order or informal basis.

Meanwhile the old mental hospitals were proving to be too large, dilapidated and unwieldy for modern psychiatric needs. Because of improved treatment, the setting up of Day Hospitals, the more enlightened and tolerant attitude of people to mental illness, and the provisions of the 1959 Act authorizing local health authorities to provide residential accom-modation and care for the mentally disabled—alas, far from satisfactory—the rate of discharge from mental hospitals increased. A survey carried out in 1961 suggested that the need for psychiatric hospital beds would fall from 3.3 per thousand of the population in 1961 to 1.8 per thousand by 1976. It was suggested therefore that part or all of many of the old mental hospitals could be closed, and indeed dates for their closure were decided upon, often prematurely it now seems.

The Department of Health and Social Security sees the needs of specific populations being served by District General Hospitals, within which are Departments for the mentally ill. Such Departments will include day-patient and out-patient services, and facilities for psycho-geriatric assess-ment. It is hoped that ultimately they will be able to replace the large mental hospitals, provided they are backed up by adequate community services. The key to the successful development of such a comprehensive service lies in the concept of the 'therapeutic team', and adequate accom-modation and community resources. A team consists of a consultant psychiatrist and his staff of nurses, occupational therapists and social workers, responsible for a population of about 60 000. The aim is to provide a flexible service, and whenever possible to treat the patient in the com-munity. A good relationship between members of the team, family doctors, district nurses, health visitors, and local authority social workers is essential. The concept is an exciting one which will call for new skills and initiative from nurses.

MENTAL ILLNESS

Mental illness can be considered from subjective or objective points of view. The patient himself may say that he is ill, that he suffers from intoler-able anxiety and fears which seriously interfere with his life. Another patient may believe himself to be sane and rational yet his friends consider him to be mad. For instance, a man was sure that he was being watched, followed, talked about in newspapers, television and radio. The man was a manual worker, holding no position of importance in the community. Had he been a leading political or business figure, or a member of the Royal family, his beliefs might have been accepted by many people as perhaps reasonable. As it was, because his ideas were so bizarre in relation to his social and cultural background, he was considered to need psychiatric treatment. In recent years the idea that such people are mentally ill has been criticized. Rather, it is said, the patient's family or society should be considered to be 'ill'. Such an extreme view is generally looked upon as untenable, but it has led to greater awareness of the interactions that go on between a patient and his relatives, and the fact that he is often forced into the role of scapegoat.

It is impossible to evaluate a patient fully without understanding his social and cultural background. Nonetheless extreme forms of mental illness, schizophrenia and psychotic depression, severe subnormality and dementia, are recognizable in any culture, even though we may not understand how or why they develop and what social stresses are responsible. Schizophrenic illnesses occur throughout the world, as much in backward as in developed countries. The current work on the International Pilot Study of Schizophrenia suggests that the main symptoms of schizophrenia are recognizable whatever a patient's race and nationality.

In a developing country such as, say, Nigeria, where psychiatric facilities are limited, particularly in rural areas, only severely ill patients whose behaviour will no longer be tolerated by the community, are admitted to mental hospitals and treated. In the U.K. nearly all new cases of schizophrenia are admitted initially to a psychiatric hospital or unit.

Psychiatry is concerned with the study and treatment of mental illness and disordered mental processes; these in turn may produce physical disorders. Increasingly, as social conditions and the overall physical health of the population have improved, so paradoxically has the demand for medical treatment risen. Symptoms which 50 years ago would have been accepted stoically, are now brought to the doctor to investigate and treat. The number of prescriptions for psychotropic drugs rises steadily, as does the amount of sickness and absence from work.

Medicine, of which psychiatry is a part, has reached a crossroads. No longer is it possible to ignore a patient's social problems and psychiatric state. Epidemiological studies suggest that at least 20 per cent of patients present with 'conspicuous psychiatric morbidity', although this is not infrequently overlooked by doctors. This is largely because the patient expresses his symptoms in strictly physical terms, physical illness still having greater social acceptance. In addition, many psychosomatic conditions such as asthma, dermatitis, colitis, are strongly influenced by emotional states.

It is essential to understand that psychiatric patients are ill, not simply 'lacking in moral fibre', and that they need and will benefit from treatment. Some nurses find this difficult to accept and are resentful, hostile and frightened when they first come into contact with psychiatric disorders.

Few maintain these feelings once they get to know a patient and understand his symptoms.

Psychiatric disorders are widespread, and psychiatric patients occupy nearly half the National Health Service hospital beds in the country. It is estimated that about one woman in fifteen and one man in twenty are likely to need psychiatric treatment in hospital at some time in their lives, and that one family out of every five will contain someone with psychiatric illness.

CAUSES OF MENTAL ILLNESS. All mental illness and psychiatric symptomatology develops from the interaction of a person's personality with one or more stresses. The stress may be 'internal', the result of organic and physiological changes within the body (uraemia, deficiency diseases, endocrine disturbances, carcinoma, vascular changes, intoxicants, and so on) or 'external'.

It is important to recognize that external stress is not necessarily bad and to be avoided. We require continual stimulation from our environment to function efficiently. Freud saw the ideal state of mind as a lack of tension, but this is only possible and desirable with death. It is impossible to have life without stress, which is only another way of saying that everyone has to adapt continually. Without stress there would be no stimulation and therefore no development. Young children go out of their way to seek stimulation. Watch how a small child continually explores and experiments with his environment. This is essential for the growth of his mental functions, and children who are overmothered and protected from stress are less able to fend for themselves in later life.

But on the other hand stress can be overwhelming. In a young child overwhelming stress can retard one or more aspects of his mental development seriously. What and where and when it is overwhelming depends partly on constitutional factors and on previous experiences. There are probably critical ages for the development of different functions, and whether or not stress has an adverse effect may depend on the age of the child at the time. For instance, there is some evidence that the stress caused by separating a child of under five from his mother for more than three months may, in some cases, retard his emotional development and warp his personality.

Perhaps it is helpful to think of stress in terms of physics. Stress then refers to any force exerting pressure on an object. The internal reaction of the body to the stress is known as *strain*. The nature and extent of the strain depends on the material of the body and on the way in which it is constructed. Thus different bodies show strain in different degrees and in different ways. Stress is tolerated up to a certain level. Beyond that level there is a danger that the stress will prove too much for the body to withstand. Consider, for example, a boiler which can only function efficiently above a certain pressure of steam. But if the safety valve sticks and the pressure goes on increasing inside, sooner or later the boiler will explode.

A similar state of affairs exists in the human body. Individual personality depends partly on inheritance and partly on past experience. Thus it is both heredity and environment that determine how much stress and of what kind any one person can deal with. If you have successfully overcome an attack of measles in childhood you will usually have no difficulty in dealing with future infections. This is because your body will have 'learned' to produce antibodies to the virus. During the first attack the body learnt to adapt and so to deal with future stress of this type. In a similar way a person learns to deal with emotional situations later in life. Defences are developed during early experiences and these are repeated whenever similar situations arise.

Individuals vary enormously in what is and is not stressful to them. Just how stressful any situation or event is depends on its special significance to that person. Some situations are very stressful for most people, for example a serious road or rail accident. Some situations affect a few people much more than others. The sudden death of an ancient mother probably causes some natural grief in all her children; but the unmarried daughter may be increasingly distressed and eventually may even become psychiatrically ill. An examination failure may have little effect on one nurse, whereas in another it may precipitate a breakdown because her self-esteem depends on her doing well and gaining public acclaim. The death of a cat is not likely to be a serious tragedy in a happy family, but a lonely old lady may collapse when her cat dies.

Stress also occurs on a mainly physical level. Starvation, thirst, injury, physical illness, and extremes of heat and cold may cause direct damage to the body, or bring about changes which may interfere with its efficient functioning. If the stress is too great the homeostasis mechanisms break down and death may occur.

The effect of overwhelming psychological stress on the nervous system is to cause it to become unstable and maladaptive. Indecision and emotional liability may appear in someone who was previously decisive and stable. A soldier who is overwhelmed by fear may run straight towards the enemy guns instead of taking cover. A wife who has just seen her husband killed before her eyes may laugh and joke as though nothing has happened. A girl who is assaulted may try to shout but may lose her voice. In some instances the whole personality disintegrates and schizophrenia appears. It is these extreme reactions to stress that are the concern of psychiatrists.

There is increasing interest in a possible relationship between the occurrence of stressful events in a person's life and the development of physical or mental disease. Studies have shown that bereavement is followed by increased psychiatric morbidity and mortality (see p. 66). The onset of acute schizophrenia is often immediately preceded by considerable stress. Stressful events precede the onset of depressive illness, although they usually extend over a longer period of time. During a war or revolution, psychiatric morbidity among the combatants is directly related to the physical casualty rate and therefore the physical danger encountered.

Sometimes it seems that psychiatric disorders follow immediately from the stressful event, for instance after childbirth or hysterectomy. In other instances psychiatric disorder emerges into the open only after months or even years have passed. We still do not know how stress brings about mental and physical disease, although Selye's general adaptation syndrome may provide a partial explanation. Nor do we know whether the stress acts merely as a non-specific precipitant to the illness, or has a more specific effect by linking up with and bringing forward earlier conflicts and disturbances.

The most common stresses today are:

1. *Loss of family or social cohesion.* Bereavement has already been discussed. Loss of a parent, particularly a mother, in early childhood, predisposes to depression in later life. Bereavement in middle age is liable to be followed by depressive illness and increased risk of coronary thrombosis. Divorce and separation, the break up of a family, retirement from work, are all liable to be followed by depression and suicide. Until the mid-fifties, single women are more prone to commit suicide than married women or men, presumably because of their way of life and relative isolation.

A marriage which to an outsider may appear to be an unhappy one is not necessarily stressful. An aggressive husband with a 'masochistic' wife who seeks punishment compulsively, may have frequent quarrels but these are probably necessary to keep the marriage together. On the other hand, frequent and violent quarrelling is known to be very stressful to the children. In time the original psychological needs of one partner for the other are liable to change. The arrival of a child often alters a marital relationship. One or other of the partners may become involved in an extra-marital affair. Suppressed resentments over a long period can bring about intolerable tensions and depression. A woman trapped in an unwanted marriage by a child whose birth was resented, an unmarried daughter supporting and living with a cantankerous old mother, may both eventually break down and require psychiatric treatment.

Bad housing and overcrowding have adverse effects on physical and mental health. But moving to a new and more satisfactory home is not necessarily advantageous. Strange surroundings, unfriendly neighbours, create an increasing sense of isolation which can be extremely stressful. The concept of 'suburban neurosis' among people, especially women, who move from a central city area to a peripheral housing estate, was described in 1938. This was then attributed to the loss of familiar surroundings, social isolation, distance from employment and high expenses. Although the relationship between the social conditions of new housing estates and neurotic disorders has recently been questioned, such a situation is undoubtedly stressful to some people. For a long time it has been recognized that immigrants have a considerably higher than average risk of developing psychiatric disorders. Immigrants to this country, particularly when coloured, have to contend with considerable stresses, although these are often cushioned by the presence of their families and friends. Bad housing is an additional stress for the immigrant, but many will not seek help for psychiatric symptoms until severely ill.

2. *Stresses concerning finances and work.* Financial stresses may be real, 'imaginary' (reflecting an insecure personality), or more often a mixture of both. A man may have to save or spend excessively in order to 'keep up appearances' or to maintain children at private schools beyond his financial means. Most people are distressed to lose their job. Not only finances but morale and self-respect suffer. But relatively few people actually break down if they are sacked or demoted. Those people who do are insecure, constantly needing to bolster themselves up with success and praise. They are limited in ability, but because they may be conscientious and hardworking they sometimes reach positions of responsibility beyond their capacity. Sooner or later they break down.

Another type of patient has great drive and ability. At first fantasy and reality intertwine. Success follows success and suddenly he finds himself in charge of a large organization and there seems no reason why he should not continue to expand. But he is unable to delegate responsibility, cannot trust anyone else to do a job properly. Bogged down by detail, he becomes increasingly exhausted. Anxiety mounts and suddenly explodes into panic attacks.

PSYCHIATRIC CLASSIFICATION

A classification of disease requires an understanding of its causes. Pneumonia a century ago was a syndrome, a group of symptoms indicating disease of the lung. Today the pneumonias are clearly classified on an aetiological basis. Psychiatry, unfortunately, is still in the syndrome stage. Our understanding of the aetiology of psychiatric disorders is still rudimentary, although growing. The classification of psychiatric disorders is therefore bound to be unsatisfactory. Yet a classification is necessary if psychiatrists are to anticipate the outcome of any illness, and to research and communicate with one another.

A syndrome is made up of a number of symptoms which, when grouped together, form a recognizable pattern. It is important to understand that a disorder such as schizophrenia is a syndrome and not an aetiological entity. Schizophrenia was first identified as a syndrome by Emil Kraepelin (1856–1926) under the name 'dementia praecox'. Just over a decade later, Eugene Bleuler (1857–1939) suggested the term schizophrenia instead. Unlike Kraepelin he believed that the disease sometimes remitted and did not invariably cause serious deterioration of the personality. Today, in an attempt to narrow the syndrome of schizophrenia and to gain greater diagnostic agreement among psychiatrists, Kurt Schneider's concept of 'first rank' symptoms is often used. But only when a biochemical basis for the schizophrenias is discovered will their classification become really satisfactory.

NEUROSIS AND PSYCHOSIS. It is still customary to use these terms, although it is often difficult to make a clear distinction. A patient with a neurosis recognizes that he is ill, although he may not connect his symptoms with an obvious emotional conflict. Only *part* of his personality is involved and he remains in contact with reality, able to recognize the subjective quality of his symptoms and to distinguish between 'me' and 'not me'. The psychotic patient on the other hand has his entire personality distorted by his illness. He accepts his symptoms as real, and out of them he reconstructs his environment, recreates a world which only he can recognize; he is followed by strangers, rays are directed at him, women are secretly having intercourse with him, unknown voices criticize him, and so on. No amount of talk will persuade him to change his mind.

While the neurotic can continue to adapt socially, the psychotic cannot and is no longer capable of continuing his work or even of living with his family. Indeed, his sense of self-preservation is seriously disturbed. An acute schizophrenic or severely depressed patient can be seen to be psychotic and in need of treatment. But such a patient may retain insight to some degree, recognize that he is ill and seek treatment himself. On the other side of the coin, a neurotic patient sometimes appears to be incapable of distinguishing between his fantasy world and what is real, and is as incapable of adapting to society as a psychotic patient.

The neuroses are usually separated from *personality disorders*. Again the distinction is in many ways an artificial one since the neuroses may co-exist with a disordered personality. A neurotic patient suffers from his symptoms, while the patient with a personality disorder is more likely to make other people suffer. The term *vulnerable* personality implies that a patient reacts excessively to relatively mild stress.

ORGANIC AND FUNCTIONAL PSYCHOSES. Anything which interferes with the normal functioning of the brain is likely to cause changes in behaviour. Acute confusional states (delirium) and chronic organic states (dementia) arise from many causes. The term *functional* psychosis refers to manic depression and schizophrenia, the basic causes of which are still not known.

THE PSYCHIATRIC EXAMINATION

The psychiatric examination aims at collecting as much information as possible about the patient, in order that the different factors contributing to the patient's breakdown can be evaluated.

It is important to put the patient at his ease, and gain his confidence and co-operation. It is best to let him tell his own story at first, without unnecessary interruption. Good interviewing is probably an art, but something of it can be learnt. The good interviewer must know what information to draw out of his patient. He must not be over-anxious himself, and above all he must have the capacity to listen and observe, for good interviewing involves both verbal and non-verbal communication. The way a patient behaves during his history, when and where he pauses or obviously avoids certain topics, when he blushes or shows strong emotions, are important clues to the patient's problems. The first psychiatric interview is not only of diagnostic value but is often highly therapeutic, particularly if the patient feels himself liked and understood by the interviewer.

Whenever possible, the patient's account should be verified from a close relative or friend. This is sometimes done by a psychiatric social worker (P.S.W.) or domiciliary nurse, who may visit the patient's home.

FAMILY HISTORY. It is necessary to find out whether any blood relative, on either side of the family, has had any form of breakdown, killed himself, drunk excessively, been in prison or in a mental institution. Patients are sometimes reluctant to reveal family skeletons. Thumb-nail sketches of the parents and the home atmosphere should be obtained. A *predisposition* to functional psychoses such as manic depression and schizophrenia is inherited. The risk of the child of one schizophrenic parent developing schizophrenia is 1 in 15, compared to just over 1 in 100 in the general population. If both parents have had schizophrenia, the chances rise to more than 1 in 2. It is important to remember that it is *predisposition* to the disease which is inherited. Certain environmental stresses must also be present before signs and symptoms of the disease appear. Even when one of a pair of identical twins develops schizophrenia, the other escapes in 20 per cent or more of cases. As they have similar genes the differences must be in their environments.

There is less evidence about the way *neurotic illnesses* are inherited, although they are certainly more common in some families than in others. The relative roles of nature and nurture in psychiatric illness are still disputed, but the arguments are futile. Neurotic individuals are not likely to make satisfactory parents, to be able to give their child the stability and security he needs. Whether or not a predisposition to break down is inherited, therefore, neurotic parents are more likely than stable parents to produce neurotic offspring. Broken homes, constant quarrels, desertion or absence of a parent, are common findings in the history of psychiatric patients, and should always be explored. The death of a parent during the early childhood of a patient may predispose him to depressive illness in later life.

Inquire about the patient's *birth order*. Each child plays his special individual part in the family. Inevitably, often unknowingly, parents treat each child slightly differently. First and last born, and only children, often have a particularly close relationship to their mother. The larger the family the less attention each child receives. This is more than compensated for by the sense of security existing in large families. Neurotic reactions are less common in members of large families. Adopted and illegitimate children are likely to encounter particular problems (see p. 49).

THE PATIENT'S PAST HISTORY

BIRTH WEIGHT AND DELIVERY. INFANCY. Prematurity, a history of foetal distress, birth injury or jaundice may be factors in mental subnormality. (See Separation Anxiety, p. 50.)

Information about breast-feeding usually has to be obtained from the patient's mother. Whether fed with breast or artificial milk is probably of no importance in itself. But breast-fed babies tend to be handled more than bottle fed babies and tactile stimulation seems to influence emotional development in infancy. The mother's attitude to the infant may be revealed by her account of the child's feeding habits. A mother who satisfactorily breast-fed for six months or more is unlikely to be rejecting or over-anxious.

Feeding difficulties, severe constipation or constant bouts of sickness in the child's early years, suggest that his mother may have been over-anxious and worried. Sometimes everything seems to have gone well for the first three or four years. Then the mother again becomes pregnant, or she or the child have to spend some weeks in hospital, away from home. After this the child's behaviour becomes difficult.

Many so called 'neurotic traits', such as nail-biting, tics, food fads, tantrums and sleep-walking, are so common in children as to mean nothing except in relation to total behaviour. Bed-wetting, in boys especially, may go on until six or seven or even later. There is however a strong relationship between persistent antisocial behaviour in childhood and later behaviour disorders.

PROGRESS AT SCHOOL. This is a rough guide to the patient's level of intelligence. Arithmetic is particularly difficult for anyone of below average intelligence. A few children have great difficulty in learning to read, a condition known as *dyslexia*. In a proportion of these, emotional factors may be responsible for the backwardness. A vicious circle often occurs, increasing emotional disturbances and making reading still more difficult.

Serious reading retardation is present in about 4 per cent of seven year old children in the U.K., excluding those with severe subnormality. There is a strong link between reading retardation and delinquency. Childhood ambitions are sometimes revealing. Children who lack self-confidence may set themselves unrealistically high targets; others aim too low in order not to have to admit failure.

OCCUPATION. A person's work record often indicates his stability and perseverance. After leaving school young people may change jobs frequently before finding what they want. But the person who goes on changing his job, never staying anywhere for longer than a year or so, usually has little ability to withstand every day tensions and frustrations.

Puberty is a time of change and adjustment. Attitudes to parents, sexual attitudes and relationships, ways of dealing with sexual tensions, moral and social behaviour, will reveal the level of maturity attained and show up unresolved conflicts and feelings of guilt. Discussion of the patient's sexual behaviour or marriage often shows how well he can adapt himself in this respect. Conflicting loyalties to his parents and wife may underlie complaints of impotence, depression, or alcoholism. Pregnancy, the menopause and retirement are stressful and sometimes difficult periods, calling for considerable readjustment.

A study of *past health* should include not only major illnesses, but minor symptoms which have resulted in time off work. In childhood, long periods of absence from school for minor illness may reflect an over-protective, anxious mother. In adult life, frequent absenteeism is often a sign of emotional disturbance. If there have been previous psychiatric breakdowns, knowledge of their symptoms, duration, and response to treatment may suggest how long the present symptoms will last and the type of treatment to give.

The personality before the outset of symptoms must be carefully assessed. A patient's account of himself may be misleading. A depressed man may describe himself as a monster of depravity; an inadequate psychopath may paint a grandiose picture of himself. Neither account will tally with what each has done with his life or what friends and relatives say about him.

Questions of the following sort are helpful in the assessment:

(*Cyclothymia*)
> Do you swing easily and for little reason from the height of joy to the depths of despair?

(*Anxiety*)
> Do you always tend to anticipate and fear the worse? Do you worry for days or weeks beforehand over an important test or encounter?

(*Schizoid*)
> Do you usually prefer your own company to that of others?
> Are you moved emotionally mainly only by non-human events and encounters?

(*Obsessive*)
> Do you have to check and recheck to an unnecessary degree your work, that you have locked doors, switched off taps and put out lights?
> Are you exceptionally upset by an unexpected change of routine in your working life?

(*Paranoid*)
> Do you feel that people try to do you down all the time?
> Are you treated unjustly at work?

(*Hysterical*)
> Do you feel that people always let you down eventually, and that no one quite comes up to your standards?
> Do you like to be the centre of attention at any gathering?

(*Hypochondriacal*)
Do you worry continuously about your bodily health, perhaps of one part in particular?

HISTORY OF THE PRESENT ILLNESS. Ask the patient when he last felt really well. This will tell you the approximate time of onset of the present illness. Then inquire about possible precipitating factors.

Not all patients are co-operative. Some may insist that there is nothing wrong with them, that they have been made to attend under false pretences. Some will say that it is their spouse who is ill. On occasions husband and wife may accuse one another, and it then becomes apparent that both are mentally ill. Some degree of *folie à deux* is not at all uncommon.

A history cannot be obtained from a patient whose consciousness is seriously disturbed, or who is stuporous or grossly overactive and distractible. All that can then be done is to record behaviour and talk, and carry out a physical examination.

Physical examination should be done as soon as possible. Cerebral neoplasms, endocrine disorders, renal and liver failure, disseminated sclerosis, and so on may present with psychiatric symptoms. The patient's behaviour during the examination may be revealing.

The body build should be recorded. There is a rough correlation between a patient's body build and the form of mental illness he develops. *Manic depressive* illness tends to occur in *pyknic* or *endormorphic* people, *schizophrenia* in those of *asthenic* or *ectomorphic* build. If schizophrenia does occur in someone of pyknic build the chances of recovery are increased. Conversely, depression in an asthenic individual sometimes has a schizophrenic colouring.

EXAMINATION OF THE MENTAL STATE

APPEARANCE AND BEHAVIOUR. The facial expression, neatness of dress, speed of movement and speech, and attitude towards other people are quickly noticed. A hypomanic patient is over-active, over-talkative, constantly interrupting, impatient and often amusing. Obsessional patients often try to control the interview and clearly reveal the conflict they have between obedience and defiance. They repeat the examiner's questions, perhaps treat the most banal remark as a pearl of wisdom, ask him to define his questions more clearly, glance at their watch, produce long written lists of symptoms and questions. Characteristically they arouse both boredom and irritation in the interviewer. The hysterical personality patient is at the opposite pole to the obsessive. Difficult and child-like in behaviour as the hysteric may at times be, he is never dull. A depressed patient may be dressed carelessly. His movements and speech are slow and his face is fixed in a mask-like expression of misery. This is known as *retardation*. A dementing patient may or may not be untidy, depending on the care of others. He is often slow, inattentive, puzzled. If pressed too hard he will collapse like a child, in what is known as a 'catastrophic reaction'. A schizophrenic may smile fatuously and make strange gestures and grimacings; or he will advance cautiously into the room, looking suspiciously about him before sitting down. He may be negativistic, refusing to co-operate or speak (*mutism*).

DISORDERS OF MOOD AND EMOTION. (*Affect* is often used in place of mood.) Some anxiety is shown by most patients at the first interview, whatever the complaint. Tense muscles, constantly fidgeting hands, and clammy skin are easily recognized. Total absence of anxiety is one of the hallmarks of hysteria; some schizophrenics also show noticeable lack of concern.

Agitation occurs when anxiety overflows into motor activity. The patient cannot keep still. He continually paces the floor, wringing his hands and muttering aloud to himself. Agitation is particularly likely to occur during *involutional depression*.

Depression is usually obvious from the general air of gloom and despondence, although 'smiling depression' is seen from time to time. There is a marked contrast between depression and the infectious gaiety and over-activity of *mania*. Suicidal ideas should always be asked about openly.

Flattening of affect occurs in schizophrenia, resulting in apathy and lack of emotional response. *Rapport*, that indefinable feeling of being 'on the same wavelength', is absent. Talking to a schizophrenic is sometimes likened to having a pane of glass inserted between you and the patient.

Splitting of affect is also characteristic of schizophrenia and describes the divergence between mood and thought. This causes *incongruity of affect*. For instance, a patient giggled most of the time as he described how his beloved mother had died of cancer. Ecstatic states are sometimes experienced by schizophrenics, and the patient feels a sense of exaltation, of mystical possession and rapture. It differs from the elation of hypomania in that it is not associated with over-activity and flight of ideas.

Depersonalization and *derealization* describe feelings that everything has altered and become shadowy and unfamiliar, as though seen in a dream. The patient can feel no emotion of any kind. *Depersonalization* affects the individual: he himself has changed and this is why the world looks different. In *derealization* the world itself changes, not the observer. A depersonalized patient said, 'This is not my body,' although she knew intellectually that it was. The everyday feelings of familiarity had been lost. These conditions can occur in various disorders, but are particularly common in depression, phobic anxiety and obsessional illness.

Déjà vu is an inexplicable feeling of familiarity, of having 'been here before', not necessarily abnormal.

DISORDERS OF PERCEPTION. What we perceive is influenced by our interests, needs and emotions. A man in the desert who is parched with thirst sees water in place of the sun's reflection off the sand. A shipwrecked sailor mistakes the crest of a wave for land. Misinterpretation of a sensation is known as an *illusion*. *Illusions* are conspicuous during states of confusion and fear. A *delirious* patient mistakes fluff on her bed for insects. A frightened man sees the post at the foot of his bed as a menacing shape looming out of the darkness.

Hallucinations differ from illusions in that no external stimuli are necessary. Mental images arise spontaneously within the brain and are projected to the outside world as though real.

Hallucinations need to be distinguished from dreams. Hypnogogic and hypnopompic hallucinations are experienced by many people as they are about to fall asleep or when waking up. The commonest hallucinations are auditory, usually hearing your name called; then come visual hallucinations. They are of no significance on their own. In schizophrenia the characteristic hallucinations are auditory, repeating a patient's thoughts, or criticizing and abusing him. Visual hallucinations are more typical of acute organic and confusional states. Visual hallucinations occur in schizophrenia but are not of primary diagnostic value in that condition. They occur in hysteria and in epilepsy, particularly involving the temporal lobe. Lilliputian hallucinations, the patient seeing tiny people (*micropsia*), occur in temporal lobe epilepsy. Tactile hallucinations are experienced in confusional states and sometimes by drug addicts. A cocaine addict may feel animals crawling under his skin (*formication*). Schizophrenics sometimes report hallucinations of touch, and some middle-aged female depressives complain of bizarre sensations around their genitalia. Hallucinations of smell occur in organic conditions, particularly temporal lobe epilepsy, schizophrenia and psychotic depression. So also with hallucinations of taste.

DISORDERS OF THINKING. Thought processes, as well as bodily movements, become slow in depression. This is known as *retardation*. Retardation may be so pronounced as to amount to *stupor*. All activity is reduced to a minimum, but consciousness is not affected. Remarks made near a stuporous patient are remembered by him and may later prove embarrassing. Stupor also occurs as a result of schizophrenia and other conditions.

Thought processes become accelerated during *mania*. One idea rapidly suggests another, and the stream of continuous talk changes frequently (*flight of ideas*). But there is always some connection between the changes, unlike the sometimes rapid but disconnected talk of the schizophrenic. Manic patients are *distractible* and rarely stick to one idea for long. Sometimes the flow of thoughts is so great that speech becomes incoherent. *Pressure of thoughts* amounting to incoherence can also occur in schizophrenia. The schizophrenic may be unable to maintain his train of thoughts because of *thought blocking*. Mental processes are split and fragmented, with the result that thoughts suddenly stop and the schizophrenic's mind goes blank. Association of one idea with another may be impossible for the observer to follow, resulting in the knight's move type of thinking. Most characteristic of all in schizophrenia is over-inclusion of thought and talking past the point.

Ideas of reference are *delusional beliefs* that certain external events are specifically concerned with the patient. Atomic bomb tests, broadcasts, road repairs, a change of postman, may be felt to have some special and personal significance. Delusions may arise from attempts on the part of the patient to rationalize his abnormal sensations. He may come to believe that his neighbour is interfering with his thoughts and preventing him from thinking. These are known as *secondary delusions*. *Primary* or *autochthonous* delusions arise from 'out of the blue'. They are invariably a sign of *schizophrenia*. The start of a schizophrenic illness was a sudden 'blinding revelation' to the patient that he had a divine mission. All *delusions* are false beliefs, absurd in the light of the patient's intelligence and background, which fail to respond to reason. They occur in organic and psychotic disorders.

Delusions are not uncommon in psychotic depression. Such patients have delusions of guilt, that they are wicked sinners and have ruined their family. Nihilistic delusions also develop, the patient believing that his mind or even his body has ceased to exist. Delusions of poverty and of ill health are common. However, hypochondriacal delusions can arise in almost any condition.

Certain thoughts may preoccupy the mind to the exclusion of everything else. When such preoccupations are recognized to be unreasonable, but persist in spite of every effort to suppress them, they are known as *obsessions*. The realization that the thought, or its persistence, is absurd indicates that the patient has *insight*; contrast this with the lack of insight of patients holding delusional beliefs.

Perseveration is most characteristic of organic brain disease. The patient's pattern of behaviour and thought continues far longer than is necessary. Some perseveration sometimes occurs in normal people when tired. Perseveration needs to be distinguished from stereotypy, which occurs in catatonic schizophrenia and may be associated with verbal perseveration. *Echolalia* is the repetition of a word or a phrase spoken to the patient. *Echopraxia* is the imitation of someone's actions or part of them. They occur in catatonic schizophrenia, and are often associated with automatic obedience and *waxy flexibility*. Echolalia and echopraxia also occur in dementia.

DISORDER OF MEMORY. Memory is made up of *learning*, which requires the patient's *attention, retention, recall* and *recognition*. Memory may be affected at any or all of these stages:

(a) Any disturbance of the level of consciousness, marked distractibility and inattention will obviously interfere with memory. Sudden transitory disturbances of memory occur in epileptic seizures and post-concussional states.

(b) *Retention* is impaired in the *Korsakov syndrome*. The patient cannot retain recent happenings, although events long past may be clearly recalled. Patients sometimes compensate for this type of memory deficiency by *confabulation*, filling in the gaps with fabrications.

(c) *Recall* of past memories may be affected by strong emotion.

Overwhelming anxiety may result in a patient developing an hysterical *amnesia*, or loss of memory. A *fugue* is loss of memory in a patient who has wandered off. That retention is unaffected is shown by the ease with which memory can be restored in such cases (see p. 115).

Tests of memory from a practical point of view are divided into relatively recent and later events. Recent memory is particularly likely to be impaired in the early stages of dementia and brain damage. In progressive states of dementia loss of memory extends increasingly far back.

DISORDERS OF CONSCIOUSNESS AND INTELLIGENCE. A patient may be disorientated and be unable to say where he is or what he has been doing recently. This may be due to delirium or dementia or hysteria.

Delirium is a state of confusion, usually of sudden or sub-acute onset, with full or varying degrees of recovery. Delirium tremens for instance may terminate with full recovery of memory and intellectual functions, or may be succeeded by the Korsakov syndrome.

Dementia is a state of permanent and often progressive intellectual impairment. Memory is always affected. Emotions become unstable and the finer aspects of a patient's personality give way to selfishness and egocentricity.

Subnormality means that the person has, and always has had, an intelligence well below average.

Some simple tests, taking the patient's social and intellectual background into consideration, will provide further information.

TESTS OF ORIENTATION. Ask the patient his name, address, where he is and where he came from, how long he has been in hospital, time of day and date.

TESTS OF IMMEDIATE MEMORY. (a) Test the memory span for digits, i.e. ask him to repeat 791368. The average adult can retain at least six digits forwards, four digits backwards.

(b) Ascertain whether the patient can retain a telephone number for at least three minutes. Make sure he understands the question by asking him to repeat at once the number you give him. Carry on with the examination and then ask him for the telephone number three minutes later.

(c) Can he learn the *Babcock sentence*? 'One thing a nation must have to become rich and great, is a large supply of wood.' Adults of average intelligence can usually reproduce this sentence after one or two repetitions unless very anxious or lacking motivation. A dementing patient may require ten or more tries.

(d) Test ability to reproduce the gist of a short story with a moral. A simple one is of the donkey and the sponges. 'A donkey, laden with bags of salt, stumbled and fell as he was crossing a river. He lay in the cool water for several minutes and when he got up was surprised to find that his load was much lighter. Next day he repeated the journey, this time laden with sacks of sponges. Thinking to lighten his load, he lay down in the river but when he tried to rise the load was so heavy that his back was broken and he drowned.' After the patient has been asked to reproduce the story he

94

should then say what is signifies. He may give a literal (concrete) interpretation, suggesting mental subnormality, dementia or schizophrenia. This tests concentration and conceptual thought, as well as memory.

Another test of conception and concentration is known as 'serial sevens': subtract 7 serially from 100, i.e. 93, 86, 79, ..., 2.

GENERAL KNOWLEDGE. Questions are useful as tests of memory, and may sometimes cause the patient to reveal delusional ideas:

> Current events that have featured in the newspapers within the last few weeks.
> The present Prime Minister and his three immediate predecessors.
> Names of members of the Royal family.
> The capitals of various countries.

TESTS OF ABSTRACT THOUGHT. The short story with a moral has already been discussed above.

Ask for the meaning of a proverb, such as 'a rolling stone gathers no moss', 'people who live in glass houses shouldn't throw stones', etc.

Ask the patient to describe the differences or similarities between objects, such as apple and orange, horse and donkey, man and monkey.

TESTS OF ARITHMETICAL ABILITY. These may show up subnormality, dementia, confusion and inattention. They will obviously need to be varied for age and background. It is useful to recognize that subtraction is harder than addition, and division more difficult than multiplication.

More formal tests can be given if necessary. In *dementia*, conceptual and abstract thought is gradually replaced by literal or concrete thinking. The patient's vocabulary, however, remains intact until late. Since a man's I.Q. roughly corresponds to the size of his vocabulary, it is possible, by comparing vocabulary I.Q. with the I.Q. derived from other tests, to determine the degree of dementia.

10

PERSONALITY DISORDERS

DEFINITION. The term *personality disorder* is used in at least two different although overlapping ways. Firstly to describe those people with neurotic personality characteristics who have particular difficulty in forming satisfactory and stable relationships. Such people are liable to leave a trail of emotional disruption and misery in their wake, and to complain continually of depression and anxiety. Secondly, and more commonly in this country, the term *personality disorder* is synonymous with adult psychopathic or sociopathic disorders, those patterns of behaviour which are considered to be socially unacceptable and undesirable, and which are not accompanied by many outward signs of anxiety and other neurotic symptoms. However, there is no hard and fast separation of psychopathic from neurotic disorder, and in any one patient there may be considerable overlapping.

PSYCHOPATHIC PERSONALITIES

DEFINITION. A *psychopathic personality* is selfish and lacks foresight and feeling for others. He is unable to profit from past experience. He cannot plan ahead realistically or see the consequences of his actions. He is impulsive, like a small child, and cannot control his whims as other people do. He feels little or no sense of responsibility, of right and wrong, or remorse for what he does. Neither punishment nor kindly treatment appear to alter him. He is impulsive and liable to explosive outbursts of violence. With other people he is continually demanding, rarely giving anything in return. He seems to be incapable of any deep emotional feeling for others. Not unexpectedly, the psychopath sometimes comes into conflict with society. Perhaps because female psychopathic personalities are less likely to break the law and draw attention to themselves, psychopathy is considered to be more common among men.

HISTORY. In this country the concept of psychopathy was first used by Pritchard in 1835 in connection with *moral insanity*. As a result, psychopathy became linked with the term *moral imbecile* in the *Mental Deficiency Act* of 1913. In fact there is no relationship between intelligence and psychopathy, although subnormality and psychopathic personality can coexist in one individual. The *Mental Health Act* of 1959 separated the two conditions. In the 1959 Act, *psychopathic personality* is defined as 'a persistent disorder or disability of mind (whether or not including subnormality of intelligence) which results in abnormally aggressive or seriously irresponsible conduct on the part of the patient and requires or is susceptible to medical treatment'.

TYPES OF PSYCHOPATH. Psychopaths are described as *inadequate* or *aggressive* on the basis of their behaviour. They are also sometimes described in terms of their main personality features, like schizoid, hysterical, obsessive, or cyclothymic.

The *inadequate psychopath* lacks persistence and cannot stand on his own. He never stays in a job for long, and becomes bored and depressed by routine. Everyone else is held to blame for his misfortunes, never himself. Often he possesses considerable charm and is able to enlist sympathy and help from those he meets. But anyone trying to help him is likely to find himself drained dry of money and emotion. Women are sexually promiscuous and incapable of forming stable relationships. Swindlers and pathological liars are frequently inadequate psychopaths. They lie habitually, often without reason (*Pseudologia fantastica*), living more in a world of fantasy than reality. A number of them compensate for their inadequacies by drinking excessively or taking drugs.

The *aggressive psychopath* 'acts out' his impulses. Explosive outbursts of anger occur, often for little or no reason. Anger may be so intense that *clouding of consciousness* occurs, and what little self-control he has is lost. Brutal assaults and murders have been committed at these times. Such an outburst 'clears the air' and for a time the psychopath may feel relaxed and cheerful, but sooner or later tension increases. Sexual assaults and serious offences may occur. His total lack of social sense causes him to be a disruptive influence in any group, and he tends to be excluded. As a consequence, he and society come to regard each other as enemies.

There is no absolute distinction between these two types. The inadequate psychopath may have explosive outbursts; the aggressive psychopath may need to cling to others for support. Both are childlike in their responses and this has given rise to the idea that psychopaths are *immature*. There is some objective evidence for this view. Electroencephalographic patterns are often of an immature kind, particularly when there is much aggressiveness. And capillary blood vessels beneath the nails are of a shape that is usually found only in young children.

DIAGNOSIS.   It is useful to distinguish *psychopathic behaviour* or disorder from *psychopathic personality*. 'Vulnerable' personalities who have adjusted to a congenial environment may react to frustration and tension with psychopathic behaviour. Depression and psychotic illnesses may also release psychopathic behaviour.

CAUSES.   1. *Genetic*. Psychopathic disorders tend to run in families.

Genetic factors may predispose the personality to develop towards psychopathy under certain types of upbringing. Alternatively, genetic factors may cause delay in maturation of the central nervous system. This may interfere with the development of a 'conscience' and social training.

2. *Brain damage.* There is an increase of brain damage and epilepsy among psychopaths.

3. *Environmental factors.* These almost certainly play a major role, in the sense of providing faulty training. Many psychopaths come from unhappy homes, deprived of affection and any sense of security as children. There is a strong correlation between consistent parental quarrelling and violence and childhood antisocial behaviour and delinquency (see p. 47). And follow-up studies show clearly the link between childhood behaviour disorders and later psychopathic disorders. But it would be very wrong to label a child or young adolescent as a psychopath. The diagnosis should not be made readily and rarely under the age of 20.

PROGNOSIS. Psychopaths are most commonly met in early adult life. Although people frequently declare that psychopathy is incurable, the fact remains that this condition often does improve with age, under the influence of a reliable, steady relationship. Individual psychopaths may suddenly 'mature' and become responsible beings. But there is an increased mortality from suicide and accidents, and not a few spend many years in prison.

TREATMENT. Treatment is difficult and regarded by some as ineffective. A patient may refuse treatment on the grounds that he is not ill. Admitted to a conventional psychiatric hospital or unit he is usually a disruptive influence through his habit of 'acting out' with the other patients or staff.

1. Special hospitals, such as Henderson Hospital at Belmont, Surrey, and psychiatric prisons like Grendon Underwood, specialize in treating psychopaths. Treatment is based on the concept of the therapeutic community, and on 'teaching' the psychopath to behave in a more responsible way to others. He is subjected to social pressures, of approval or disapproval from his fellow psychopaths. Through such criticism and interaction it is hoped he will learn to develop greater self control and toleration. In addition, by recognizing the particular stresses which precipitate his psychopathic behaviour, he can perhaps avoid these or protect himself in advance from their effects.

2. When psychopathy seems to be due predominantly to brain damage, neurosurgery can be considered, i.e. temporal lobectomy.

3. Drugs are occasionally useful. Minor tranquillizers lessen explosive outbursts, sexual outbursts can sometimes be controlled with stilboestrol.

NURSING CARE. These patients are amongst the most difficult to nurse; they resent the nurse because of the authority she represents. At one moment they appear charming and rational, and young nurses often feel a strong sense of identification with them. They are persuasive and manipulative and are particularly liable to play one nurse off against another. Psychopaths also demand a great deal of the nurse's time. Much of their disruptive behaviour results from their need to draw attention to themselves.

In order to nurse psychopathic patients with any degree of success, it is essential that the nurse be aware of their personality deficiencies, even when the patient is at his most charming. If the nurse knows that the patient feels little responsibility for what he does, she will not feel unduly discouraged when his behaviour becomes disruptive. If she recognizes that he is manipulative, she will be able to guard against being manipulated herself.

The best attitude to adopt from the nurse's point of view, and in the interests of her patient, is one of friendly firmness. If a nurse becomes angry when she feels her patient has misbehaved and let her down in some way, she will have reacted in the way the patient intended. On the other hand she should make it clear to the patient that his behaviour is unacceptable to her as a person. Although psychopathic patients find the equable nurse infuriating at times, it is usually this type of nurse who succeeds most in re-educating the patient into a limited degree of increased maturity.

MEDICO LEGAL. A psychopath can, under the 1959 Mental Health Act, be compulsorily detained for treatment if under twenty-one. When he teaches the age of twenty-five he must be discharged unless the responsible medical officer renews the detention order on the grounds that the patient is likely to be a danger to himself or to others.

DRUG ADDICTION OR DEPENDENCE

Because of the difficulty of defining the word 'addiction', the World Health Organisation (WHO) has recommended the use of the term 'drug dependence'. Drug dependence is sometimes qualified by the drug involved, since heroin dependence for instance is very different from amphetamine or cannabis dependence, but the usefulness of this is doubtful in view of the fact that many drug takers switch from one drug to another, depending upon their needs and what is available. It is perhaps more useful to distinguish hard drugs like narcotics, which cause serious symptoms in the drug user on withdrawal, from soft drugs such as amphetamines.

Drug dependence is the persistent or periodic excessive consumption of a drug, for non-medical purposes (although initially the drug may have been prescribed medically). There are four features which characterize drug dependence, although not all of these are necessarily present in every form of drug dependence:

1. An addict craves for his drug and becomes increasingly upset if deprived of it. He uses any means to obtain the drug.

2. The addict becomes increasingly tolerant to the drug, and has to increase the dose progressively to produce the same effects as in the beginning.

3. In many cases the addict becomes physically, as well as psychologically, dependent on the drug. Sudden stoppage of supplies results in 'withdrawal symptoms'. Prolonged use of the drug brings about physiological changes in the central nervous system which cause physical symptoms and signs when the drug is suddenly stopped. Morphine and its analogues, barbiturates, and alcohol are the drugs most likely to be associated with this.

4. Either the drug taker, society, or both will ultimately suffer.

Dependence should be distinguished from *habituation*. The majority of people who take nightly sedatives, daily laxatives or vitamin pills are *habituated* to these drugs. Physical dependence and tolerance do not develop and the dose remains constant.

INCIDENCE. A number of young people experiment with soft drugs for a time, especially cannabis, L.S.D., and amphetamines, and sooner or later lose interest in them. But some persist, or move on to hard drugs. It is probably true to say that all persistent drug takers are abnormal personalities, unable to deal with everyday tensions without support. By chance or contact with other addicts, or perhaps as a result of medical treatment, drug taking begins. Addicts are of all levels of intelligence and come from all social classes. Their home backgrounds are reasonably stable, but patients show a higher than average incidence of childhood neurotic traits. Between 12–16 per cent of delinquent boys, admitted to remand homes or detention centres, give a history of amphetamine and barbiturate abuse. Sexual promiscuity and homosexuality are common among both male and female drug takers.

Different drugs have been used at different times in different societies for their psychological effects for as long as is known; alcohol, cannabis, cocaine, opium, khat, hallucinogens, tobacco, to name but a few. In England, alcohol was greatly abused during the 18th and 19th centuries. Opium, particularly in the form of laudanum, was used increasingly from the 18th century and dependence was rife in the 19th century. Famous examples are Coleridge and de Quincey. However, laws were enacted to control the use of morphine and opium, and during the present century, until about 1961, the number of people addicted to morphine-type drugs was small. The majority of them were middle-aged or older, and many had become dependent as a result of receiving morphine during a prolonged painful illness. About 10 per cent were doctors and nurses with access to dangerous drugs.

Since 1961 there has been a rapid increase in drug dependence, almost entirely among young people. In 1960 only 94 non-therapeutic heroin addicts were known to the Home Office. By 1966 the number had risen to almost 1000. Today there are over 2000. The dangerous drugs (supplied to addicts) regulations were introduced in 1968. These transferred responsibility for the treatment of narcotic drug addicts from their general practitioners to special clinics run by psychiatrists 'licensed' by the Home Office.

Dependence on amphetamine compounds and other 'pep pills' and the barbiturates are more difficult to assess but their use is certainly much more widespread. Any drug which stimulates the brain either directly or as a result of lessening tension is liable to cause addiction. It has been estimated that for every 100 000 population, misuse of barbiturates occurs in among 1200, amphetamines among 300, cannabis up to 45, and L.S.D. up to 5. A 1968 survey of over 1000 children in six schools found that at least 4 per cent had taken drugs.

Supplies of drugs are readily obtainable by addicts, as a result of theft from pharmacies and wholesalers, through stolen prescription forms and forgeries, and registration with several doctors at once. Overgenerous prescribing by doctors is probably a further source.

TYPES OF DEPENDENCE. *Morphine-type.* (Including all opium derivatives and synthetic opiate-like drugs such as heroin, pethidine, methadone, dextromoromide, etc.). All these drugs are characterized by physical and psychological dependence and tolerance. The first experience of heroin is often unpleasant and several months usually pass before regular daily injections are self-administered. The injection produces a dreamy, detached state which lasts a few hours and is then followed by increasing distress. Thus the addict is compelled to continue the pattern.

Withdrawal symptoms start after about eight hours with anxiety, apprehension, yawning, sweating, salivation, running eyes and nose, nausea and vomiting, aching limbs, abdominal cramps and diarrhoea. After twenty-four hours there is hypertension, hyperglycaemia and spontaneous erection and ejaculation.

These patients may suffer complications; dirty needles and syringes cause abcess formation, cellulitis, thrombophlebitis, septicaemia, endo-carditis, nerve palsies, jaundice, syphilis, and occasionally malaria. Opiates do not in themselves provoke criminal activity. However the need to obtain money for further supplies may do so. Drug addicts form a special subculture from which it is difficult to break away. Members come to regard drug taking, and the rituals surrounding it, almost as a higher form of life, and they feel alienated from the rest of society.

Cocaine users develop strong psychological but no physical dependence. It is usually taken in combination with opiates, either by injection or as snuff. It produces increased energy and sexual drive, and a sense of well-being. Toxic symptoms occur if the drug is taken for long. These include paranoid and psychotic states, and a sensation of insects crawling beneath the skin (*formication*). When cocaine is taken as snuff, ulceration of the nasal mucosa eventually occurs.

Barbiturate dependence is common. Smallish doses of 200–400 mg a night probably do little harm, although the electro-encephalogram pattern of sleep is altered. Daily doses of 800 mg or more, taken for several weeks, create physical dependence and result in tremor, ataxia, slurred speech, confusion. A lethal dose may inadvertently be ingested during a state of confusion. Sudden withdrawal of the drug causes epileptic fits and sometimes delirium not unlike that occurring in alcoholism. Barbiturates are often combined with amphetamines.

Amphetamines and similar drugs (phenmetrazine, methylphenidate, diethylpropion) create a sense of euphoria and a strong psychological dependence and tolerance slowly develops. There is no physical dependence. Depression, fatigue and irritability develop after withdrawal. Amphetamines impair insight and antisocial acts may occur. Toxic psychoses develop when doses exceed 50 mg a day, resembling acute schizophrenia.

HALLUCINOGENIC DRUGS. *Lysergic acid* is the one most commonly encountered after cannabis. Psychological dependence is uncommon. Physical dependence does not occur. The psychic experience caused by the drug is frequently overvalued. 'Bad trips' occur, especially in vulnerable personalities; acute anxiety, depersonalization, and psychotic episodes may persist for months or years.

Cannabis does not create physical dependence, nor does tolerance develop. But frequent use of cannabis is liable to lead to withdrawal from social activities, apathy and inertia. Depersonalization and psychotic episodes sometimes occur. Reports that long-standing cannabis dependence causes cerebral atrophy need confirmation. There is no convincing evidence that the use of cannabis leads a person to take other drugs, except through social links.

Marihuana (hashish, hemp) is smoked in the form of 'reefers'. It is not itself addictive, but is sometimes the first step on the road to other drugs.

TREATMENT. Treatment ideally aims at complete abstinence from drugs. Drugs resulting in physical dependence are generally withdrawn slowly. Social and psychological rehabilitation subsequently plays a vital role.

Heroin dependence is best treated by substituting methadone with or without a tranquillizer, and then gradually reducing the dosage over about 10 days. The reason for this is that methadone gives far fewer withdrawal symptoms than heroin. For optimum results the patients should preferably be in hospital. Those patients who cannot be weaned off their drugs may have to be maintained on a fixed dose of heroin. Recently attempts to replace heroin by high doses of methadone have met with some success. Methadone is less a drug of dependence than heroin, and in high dosage blocks its action and therefore the addict's craving for heroin. Heroin addicts who attend casualty departments with withdrawal symptoms should be given methadone 10 mg orally or by injection. In the future, substances which block the effects of drugs are likely to become major therapeutic weapons in this field.

Once a patient has been withdrawn he must be separated from his drug-dependent group. Specialized hostels, supervision, encouragement and suitable work, individual and group psychotherapy, are important in his rehabilitation, which will take at least 2 years. Ultimately the prognosis depends on the patient's personality and motivation to remain off drugs.

Ex-drug addicts have formed communities such as Phoenix House to help the rehabilitation of patients, with promising results. *Barbiturates* must always be withdrawn slowly and substituted by one of the diazepine derivatives. Antidepressant drugs may be useful later, but care must be taken not to substitute one drug of dependence by another.

Amphetamines and cocaine can be stopped abruptly.

NURSING CARE. The nurse must seek to form a friendly relationship with her patient aimed at restoring his selfconfidence and respect. She should let him know how she expects him to behave and be positive and firm in her attitude. She must be able to recognize genuine symptoms from false ones. Particularly in the first stages of treatment, drug-dependent patients produce all kind of reasons why drugs should not be withheld, and they may resort to self-injury as a means to this end. But they may also become depressed and suicidal, and vigilant observation is always necessary.

Needless to say patients should be searched for drugs on admission, and care taken that they do not obtain drugs from other patients or visitors.

ALCOHOLISM

DEFINITION. Addiction to alcohol is analogous to other drug addictions. But its widespread incidence and the seriousness of its effects make alcohol a far more serious social problem. Taking alcohol in reasonable amounts is a beneficial and socially accepted custom in our culture. It is, therefore, not easy to define alcoholism. The World Health Organisation defines alcoholics as 'those excessive drinkers whose dependence on alcohol has attained such a degree that it shows a notable mental disturbance or an interference with their bodily and mental health, their interpersonal relations and their smooth social and economic functioning; or who show the prodromal signs of such development'. It is important to recognize that considerable differences exist in the amount of alcohol which is excessive for any one drinker and leads eventually to his losing control over his drinking. Many of us have a degree of psychological dependence on alcohol. The alcoholic's dependence is extreme. Physical dependence occurs late in alcoholism and is always an ominous sign. Many doctors are still reluctant to make a diagnosis of alcoholism because of the stigma attached to the term.

Alcoholism is a complex problem, involving not only the medical profession but magistrates, police, lawyers, clergy, welfare workers and educational authorities among others.

INCIDENCE. The World Health Organisation estimated in 1955 that there were about 350 000 alcoholics in England and Wales (11 per 1000), of whom 86 000 had mental and physical complications. And there is evidence that it is increasing, especially among young people. Alcoholism occurs at all levels of society and intelligence. The incidence is six times higher in men than women.

DIAGNOSIS. The alcoholic deceives himself as well as others about the amount of alcohol he regularly consumes openly and in secret. It is always necessary to ask how much he depends on drink, at what times of the day he drinks, whether alone or in company, if he becomes drunk, suffers from loss of memory, hangovers, and how much his work and family life are affected. The young alcoholic has a strong head for alcohol and is rarely troubled by hangovers. He enjoys drinking with others and is usually one of the last to leave a party. At this stage his dependence is largely psychological.

Tolerance for alcohol progressively develops, and the alcoholic needs increasing amounts to create the same effects. He drinks in secret before parties or meetings and keeps supplies hidden in his home and workplace. His life becomes organized around his need to drink. Family finances suffer and marital problems arise. He may attempt to control himself, and to abstain altogether for days or even weeks. But sooner or later he again takes a drink, and increasingly he finds he cannot control the amount drunk. One drink leads to another and he only stops when supplies or money are exhausted. Physical changes and dependence appear. Tolerance suddenly begins to drop, so that he now becomes drunk after only a few drinks. Tremor develops. He wakes up feeling ghastly, nauseated, shaky, unable to remember the events of the night before. He needs a drink to control withdrawal symptoms, and drinking now extends through most of the day. Personal relationships suffer, he loses his job, family life is disrupted and there is a steady social decline.

Signs of physical change now appear. His manners and habits deteriorate. Judgement, insight and memory are affected. Self-control is lost. Unless he has treatment serious mental and physical complications will supervene. The more important of these are the following:

1. *Delirium tremens.* Usually, although not invariably, follows two or three days of abstinence, the result perhaps of infection or a stomach upset. It is ushered in by tremulousness and sometimes hallucinosis. The patient is confused and frightened. Illusions, hallucinations, which are usually visual, and delusions are marked. He is restless, sweating, pyrexial, anorexic and sleepless. Dehydration and electrolyte disturbances may be profound. Pneumonia is a common complication. Delirium tremens lasts for between 1–2 weeks, but death can occur, usually in the first week.

2. *Alcoholic hallucinosis.* The occurrence of auditory hallucinations in the setting of clear consciousness, sometimes following withdrawal of alcohol, is not uncommon. Most cases resolve spontaneously in a week or so, but occasionally persist for months. Sometimes hallucinosis is followed by delirium tremens, rarely by a schizophrenic illness. (But alcoholic hallucinosis and schizophrenia are separate entities.)

3. *Paranoid states* are also relatively common in chronic alcoholics, particularly pathological jealousy towards a spouse.

4. *Korsakov syndrome.* This syndrome consists of a marked loss of memory for recent events, disorientation and confabulation. The patient sometimes cannot remember what was said or done a few seconds

beforehand. To fill in memory defects he makes up stories (*confabulation*) which are often very convincing. There are usually, but not invariably, signs of peripheral neuritis. The outlook for full recovery is poor.

5. *Wernicke's encephalopathy.* In this condition there is disorientation, associated with paralysis of ocular muscles, nystagmus, ataxia. Like the Korsakov syndrome, it is believed to be due to acute deficiency of vitamin B1, superimposed on a chronic vitamin B complex deficiency.

6. Other complications of alcoholism are *cirrhosis of the liver, peripheral neuritis, cardiomyopathy, acute pancreatitis, and impotence.*

THE CAUSE OF ALCOHOLISM

1. *Familial.* Alcoholism runs in families. 45 per cent of alcoholics have parents who are or have been alcoholics. Early experience of alcoholism, and possibly genetic factors, may be important elements therefore.

2. *Sex.* Men outnumber women by 6 to 1, but this is probably related to environmental factors rather than to constitutional differences. However, women alcoholics have a worse prognosis than men; they are less well adjusted and are prone to depression.

3. *Racial.* Alcoholism is prevalent among the Irish, rare among Jews.

4. *Social.* Although both Italy and France are wine-producing countries, alcoholism is much more prevalent in France. This is believed to be due to the fact that Italians drink mainly at mealtimes. However, the more easily alcohol is obtainable the greater the incidence of alcoholism. This was seen all too well in Hogarth's England, when a man could be drunk for one penny, dead drunk for twopence. Certain types of work, for instance brewerymen, and activities involving business entertainment, are likely to hold more than their fair share of alcoholics.

5. *Psychiatric.* Anxiety in youth, depression in middle age, and loneliness in old age are conducive to alcoholism. The incidence of depression in alcoholics, especially women, is high, and the risk of suicide much increased compared to non-alcoholics.

TREATMENT

1. *'Drying out'.* Withdrawing alcohol is ideally best carried out in hospital. This allows the alcoholic to be fully assessed, both physically and mentally, infections and vitamin deficiencies treated, and long-term treatment planned.

Delirium tremens always needs hospital admission, heavy sedation and large doses of vitamin B complex. Some authorities also recommend the routine use of anticonvulsants. The most commonly used drugs for sedation are Heminevrin, chlorpromazine and chlordiazepoxide. Paraldehyde is still used in some centres, and is effective, but has the great disadvantage of being painful when given intramuscularly, and when given orally it has a filthy taste and smell and is highly irritating to the stomach. Chlorpromazine and heminevrin given together are probably the most effective combination. Chlorpromazine increases the risk of epileptic fits but this can be reduced by adding phenytoin.

2. *Group therapy* in specialized hospital units, provided the atmosphere is optimistic and positive, is helpful.

Aversion therapy using apomorphine or painful electric shocks, followed by relaxation therapy, is useful in selected patients.

Disulphiram (Antabuse) or citrated calcium carbide (Abstem) are often effective in preventing relapse. These drugs interfere with the break down of alcohol in the body, so that toxic substances accumulate. As a result alcohol causes very unpleasant symptoms in anyone taking these drugs.

Tranquillizers should be used with caution because of the risk of creating dependence. Antidepressants are given if depression is present.

Some form of supervision or support is needed, particularly by the more vulnerable patients. Many patients derive great benefit from joining Alcoholics Anonymous, a voluntary organization run by ex-alcoholics for alcoholics. Various other voluntary bodies such as the Church of England Temperance Society and the Salvation Army, also cater for the needs of alcoholics.

3. *Treatment of the Chronic Drunken Offender.* Each day, on an average, the Courts deal with some 200 drunken offences. In the past these drunks, usually homeless, jobless, and friendless, revolved through Court, prison, drunkenness, Court, and so on, a degrading, expensive, recurring futile procedure. Now rehabilitation, instead of repeated prison sentences, is being attempted by means of detoxication centres, 'skid row' hostels.

II

NEUROTIC DISORDERS

ANXIETY STATES

DEFINITION. Most people feel anxious before an important event, or when faced with grave danger. Anxiety or fear is the natural reaction of the central nervous system at such times and serves a useful purpose, and disappears when the anxiety is removed. An *anxiety state*, on the other hand, is a continual and irrational feeling of anxiety, in the absence of any justifiable cause. The anxiety may amount to panic and interfere with mental and social functions. There is no qualitative difference between normal and pathological anxiety. (The term *anxiety hysteria* was used by Freud to signify neurotic personality conflicts. He regarded *anxiety neurosis* as arising from current sexual problems.)

INCIDENCE. Anxiety states are among the most common psychiatric disorders encountered today. About 25 per cent of patients attending a psychiatric outpatient clinic have an anxiety state. Anxiety states occur about equally in both sexes, and mostly develop either in adolescence and before thirty, or in old age. Transitory symptoms are frequent in childhood. There is no evidence for linking social class with anxiety states in this country, although in the U.S.A. anxiety states are said to be more prevalent in the upper social groups. 'Suburban neurosis', anxiety states brought about by loneliness and lack of interests and outlets among females, was described in 1938. A similar description of anxiety among women living in high flats exists, but some doubt has recently been cast on both these connections.

THE PHYSIOLOGICAL CHANGES OF ANXIETY. Sympathetic and parasympathetic activities increase, although the sympathetic predominates. The adrenal cortex and medulla are both stimulated. As a result the levels of corticosteroids and of adrenaline and noradrenaline in the plasma are increased. Adrenaline, which is more potent than noradrenaline in producing the sympathomimetic effects of anxiety, is secreted in greater quantities. Anxiety symptoms can be produced in anyone by giving them intravenous adrenaline.

Free fatty acids are released from fatty tissues by the action of adrenaline, and probably increase the risk of myocardial infarction. There is a redistribution of blood to the periphery, which perhaps accounts for the symptoms of faintness and dizziness so common in anxiety states. The increased flow of blood in the forearms of patients with anxiety states can be measured by means of a plethysmograph, and provides a useful measure of anxiety. Conductance of the skin to electrical currents depends upon sweat gland activity. Anxiety neurotics tend to have sweaty palms, and therefore lower skin conductance levels (psychogalvanic reflexes).

There is no consistent change in the E.E.G., although alpha activity is often reduced in chronic anxiety.

SYMPTOMS. Anxiety is accompanied by a feeling of tension, and by increased activity of the sympathetic, parasympathetic and endocrine systems.

CHRONIC ANXIETY. Anxiety rarely remains 'free floating', that is unattached to anything, for long. Depression, exhaustion, physical symptoms, phobias or hysterical reactions soon begin to appear, depending on the personality structure of each patient.

Symptoms vary widely. Some patients complain of a constant feeling of anxiety, a sense of impending dissolution, or fears of going mad. Concentration becomes difficult, and memory and judgement suffer. Patients feel irritable and exhausted and lose their sense of enjoyment. Libido (sexual interests) and appetite diminish and some weight loss may occur, but is rarely more than 3 kg. Sleep is disturbed, particularly getting to sleep, and dreams are vivid and unpleasant. Patients feel tired and ready to go to sleep when it is time to get up. Tachycardia, palpitations and other bodily symptoms may be prominent.

Sometimes *depression* becomes the predominating symptom and it may be difficult to decide whether the anxiety is primary or secondary to the depression.

Frequently anxiety attaches itself to particular objects or situations, which are then avoided. Specific fears of this kind are known as *phobias*. Patients sometimes complain only of the *somatic symptoms of anxiety*. They become convinced and terrified that they have a fatal or unpleasant disease, cancer, leukaemia, venereal disease. These amount virtually to hypochondriacal phobias. The most common are: pain over the heart, palpitations, breathlessness and a sense of impending dissolution, sometimes known as *cardiac neurosis* or effort syndrome. Pain may arise from any of the large muscle groups of the neck, head, back or limbs. Headache, which is most often frontal and 'like a tight band' is sometimes very painful.

Gastrointestinal symptoms include nausea and vomiting, bouts of diarrhoea and/or constipation, and abdominal pain from spasm of the colon, usually in the right iliac fossa. Gynaecological and genito-urinary symptoms are common. Fear of organic disease increases anxiety, producing a vicious circle.

Fatigue is sometimes the main symptom. Any exertion brings on palpitations, dizziness and a sense of collapse.

Some patients try to reduce their sense of anxiety by eating, and consequently becoming overweight. Others resort to excessive amounts of alcohol or sedative drugs. Sleep is occasionally increased, both in depth and duration, to such an extent that narcolepsy is suspected. Increased sexual tension may result in promiscuity.

PHOBIC ANXIETY.   This is anxiety attached to some object or situation, and makes up about 5 per cent of out-patient psychiatric referrals. It is convenient to divide phobias into four groups.

1. *Monosymptomatic phobias, i.e. single phobias.*

(a) Phobias of animals, such as spiders, cats, cows, dogs, are very common in childhood. Most children grow out of them, but in a few, mostly females, the phobias persist into adult life. They make up only about 1 per cent of phobic states and are rarely more than a nuisance.

(b) Phobias of the dark, flying, heights, water, thunder, and so on, which are acquired later in life. These monosymptomatic phobias are not associated with generalized anxiety and respond extremely well to behaviour therapy.

2. *Social phobias.* These include eating or drinking in public, picking up a glass or cup, writing in front of other people. Events which include the feared activity are avoided for fear of the patient's disgracing himself by blushing, vomiting, trembling, or in some way making an exhibition of himself. These develop in late adolescence and the early twenties and are quite common. About 60 per cent of patients are female. Generalized anxiety is not marked but social phobias are obviously more incapacitating than monosymptomatic phobias. Patients respond fairly well to behaviour therapy.

3. *Multiple phobias.* The most common and incapacitating phobia is agoraphobia. The patient is afraid of going into the street, into shops, even out of her home. Not uncommonly agoraphobia is associated with claustrophobia (fear of enclosed spaces) and other phobias. The patient is in a state of constant anxiety and suffers from attacks of panic, depersonalization, and depression of mood. Nearly 80 per cent of patients are female. Agoraphobia develops most commonly in the twenties. Response to behaviour therapy is variable, being poor in patients with frequent panic attacks. Other terms which describe this condition are 'housebound housewives', and the 'phobic anxiety depersonalization syndrome'.

4. Phobias of physical symptoms of hypochondriacal phobias, have been already described above. They are frequently secondary to depressive illness, particularly when occurring in middle age and later.

AETIOLOGY

1. *Genetic factors* play an important role. Studies suggest that about 21 per cent of patients have also had anxiety states, and a further 20 per cent have over-anxious personalities. Of course it is never easy to separate heredity from upbringing, but monozygotic twins are more concordant for anxiety states than dizygotic.

2. *Childhood factors.* To some degree anxiety is probably a learned response to childhood stresses. Anxious, inconsistent parents are liable to breed anxious children, particularly if the latter have inherited an

anxious personality. A vicious circle often develops within families, the child's anxieties stimulating parental anxiety.

3. *Personality.* Eysenck's work suggests that the personality of people with anxiety states has a high degree of introversion and neuroticism, i.e. dysthymia.

4. *Precipitating factors.* External stresses may be severe or minimal, depending upon the patient's constitution: an illicit love affair, fear of failure at work after promotion, or suppressed resentment towards a relative or spouse. An illness such as influenza, glandular fever, infective hepatitis, can precipitate an anxiety state. In young people a 'bad trip' with pot or LSD may act as a precipitant.

5. *Psychodynamics.* Anxiety develops in response to a threat: to life, self-respect, a valuable relationship, material comforts, and so on. Anxiety states in the beginning usually reflect the threatened loss (which may be more neurotic and fantasied than real) of an important relationship. However, in time the anxiety comes almost to exist in its own right. The patient constructs his life around his anxiety state and the original threatened loss often becomes irrelevant from a therapeutic point of view.

Agoraphobic symptoms are often 'used' to create an intensely dependent (and resentful) relationship with a spouse.

DIFFERENTIAL DIAGNOSIS. Anxiety may be the result of organic disease rather than the cause of physical symptoms. Thyrotoxicosis, or attacks of hypoglycaemia, are readily mistaken by the unwary for anxiety. Anxiety may be felt before a serious illness reveals itself. Anxiety is absent in essential hypertension until the patient is informed about the condition. Anxiety itself raises blood pressure, especially systolic, and not a few anxious patients are regrettably 'treated' with hypotensive drugs, often to their psychiatric detriment.

Depression is nearly always accompanied by anxiety and should always be suspected in the middle aged. Schizophrenia is often ushered in by anxiety symptoms. A patient in the early stages of dementia, before insight is lost, understandably feels anxiety and depression.

The diagnosis of an anxiety state should rest on positive evidence of an anxious and predisposed personality, and/or reasonably severe stress in the recent past.

TREATMENT

1. Acute anxiety needs immediate and heavy sedation. The longer it is allowed to persist the more difficult symptoms are to remove. Continuous narcosis may be necessary at times. Exploration under an intravenous barbiturate is sometimes valuable and may result in *abreaction* if significant material is brought to light. However, unless care is taken anxiety may be increased by this method. Heavy sedation should continue for 48 to 72 hours and then be slowly reduced.

2. The prognosis of a chronic anxiety or phobic anxiety state depends on the basic personality structure of the patient. Where this is good, and particularly when there are signs of reactive depression, symptoms often

respond rapidly to an antidepressant drug such as phenelzine (Nardil) combined with a tranquillizer. Tricyclic antidepressants also help some patients. Patients with less adequate personalities respond better to a tranquillizer alone. Drug dependence should be guarded against. Intravenous diazepam, 20–30 mg, given once or twice a week for 4 weeks, is a useful adjunct to all therapy, particularly in phobic anxiety states.

3. *Behaviour therapy* is very effective, particularly in phobic anxiety not associated with generalized anxiety. All the monosymptomatic, and many of the social phobias, respond well either to desensitization or flooding. The latter is less time-consuming and often more effective than desensitization. Agoraphobia responds less well, although behaviour therapy may be useful at some stage in combination with other treatments.

4. Psychotherapy needs to be given concomitantly with physical treatments. The mechanisms bringing about the symptoms should be explained and the patient told firmly that he has no organic disease. It is wise not to probe too deeply into the background of inadequate patients, for fear of breaking down still more their psychological defences. Both individual and group psychotherapy may be useful.

5. Where depression coexists with anxiety, electro-shock may be helpful. But great care is needed, as electro-shock is liable to make a primary anxiety state worse. In any case electro-shock should be accompanied by heavy sedation.

6. Intravenous infusion of one molar strength DL sodium lactate (5 ml/kg body weight) over about 20 minutes brings about panic and anxiety symptoms in patients with chronic anxiety. Twice weekly treatments for three weeks have produced good results on the basis of helping patients to recognize and tolerate their symptoms.

7. Prefrontal leutocomy should be considered for patients of good personality, disabled by chronic anxiety and unresponsive to all treatment. Stereotactic methods have given encouraging results.

HYSTERICAL REACTIONS

The word hysterical is used in a number of ways.

1. The term *hysterical personality* refers to an egocentric, narcissistic personality, who is often very difficult to live or work with.

2. *Hysterical behaviour* means that (a) the emotions and reactions of the person concerned are exaggerated, for instance, screaming with pain and demanding analgesics for no good reason in the view of medical staff, or symptoms are prolonged beyond the time of apparent recovery, and (b), that the patient seeks to gain something, although not necessarily consciously so, from such behaviour.

3. *Hysteria* is used to cover a huge amorphous group of conditions, predominately psychosomatic, for which no reasonable organic cause

can be found. These are better described in terms of an underlying psychiatric state: anxiety, depression, and so on. For further discussion of this group, see the section of psychosomatic disorders.

4. *Dissociative states and conversion reactions of hysteria.* As in (3) above, physical symptoms and certain mental disturbances occur in the absence of organic disease. The symptoms represent an unconscious attempt by the patient to deal with apparently unsurmountable conflicts. The patient therefore needs to be ill and there is always some gain for the patient, although to others this may seem trivial compared to the ensuing disability. Before dissociation and the onset of hysterical symptoms, the patient shows and feels anxiety. With the appearance of hysteria anxiety disappears, and the patient presents a picture of unconcern or 'belle indifférence'. A functional part of the brain has split off from consciousness and now operates in isolation.

Hysteria derives its name from the ancient belief that the disorder is due to the 'wanderings' of the uterus. But men as well as women can develop hysteria. A sexual causation has long been attributed to hysteria. Galen, who first proposed the idea of male hysteria, thought it came about from retained semen, due to sexual abstinence.

INCIDENCE. Short-lived hysterical conversions are not uncommon in childhood; blindness, paralysis of a limb, inability to speak or swallow. They occur in response to a particular stress and nearly all resolve themselves completely without treatment. Only if hysterical symptoms persist or occur frequently need they cause concern.

Hysteria as occurred throughout recorded history. It was common in the latter half of the 19th century, partly because of medical interest in the condition at that time. Today, hysterical conversion states still occur. Gross paralysis and abnormalities of gait and posture probably only develop in patients of low intelligence. Medical ignorance, isolation and fear, all increase the incidence. The incidence is much greater in primitive societies.

CLINICAL SYMPTOMS. *Symptoms* are most easily considered under separate motor, sensory and mental headings. But all types of symptoms can be seen in the same patient.

Motor. Paralysis, spasm or *contracture* of any voluntary muscle can occur. But typically, movements rather than individual muscles are affected. Testing shows inconsistencies. Reflexes are normal. Passive movement often meets with undue resistance, which can be seen to affect a wide range of musculature. However, if a hysterical paralysis lasts for several years muscle tone and reflexes will considerably diminish, and there will be some disuse, muscle atrophy and the overlying skin will be cool and cyanotic.

Tremor is usually gross, often varies and may cease if the patient's attention is drawn to something else. Abnormalities of *gait* vary from a drunken stagger to extraordinary contortions. Speech may be affected. Aphonia is rarely complete and the patient is able to whisper and cough loudly. *Stammering* is a common symptom. *Dysphagia, globus hystericus, ptosis, overbreathing* to the extent of causing alkalosis and tetany, *vomiting* and *faints* are also frequently seen.

Hysterical fits may be difficult to distinguish from *epileptic fits*. In fact epileptics may bring on true fits by hysterical overbreathing. Hysterical fits do not have the tonic/clonic phases of epilepsy. They invariably occur before an audience and may continue for half an hour or more. Attempts to restrain the patient's excessive movements lead to redoubled activity. Foaming at the mouth, wild cries and facial contortions produce a dramatic scene. Hysterics rarely harm themselves.

Sensory. Anaesthesia, blindness, deafness and loss of taste may be presenting symptoms. Some disturbance of sensation is extremely common in anxious patients and is of no significance alone.

Hysterical anaesthesia is typically of a 'glove and stocking' type of distribution corresponding to the patient's ideas rather than to any known nerve distribution. Examination often induces changes in the area of anaesthesia.

A patient may complain of blindness, yet be able to find his way to the door across a room full of obstacles. Occasionally he will complain of 'funnel' vision.

Mental. Amnesia and fugue states occur. Rarely, the patient splits into two or more separate personalities, like Dr. Jekyll and Mr. Hyde.

Amnesia, or loss of memory, occurs after a terrifying event which the patient wishes had never happened. A respectable young man fell in love with a good-time girl and stole from the petty cash in order to entertain her. He was accused of theft by his manager. Panic-stricken he ran into the street. Suddenly all memory of what he had done disappeared from consciousness and was replaced by unconcern. But so great was the *repressing force* needed to do this that other memories were also affected. In this example the young man was unable to recall his name or anything to do with his past life. He was admitted to hospital with total amnesia.

Sometimes a patient who has developed amnesia wanders far away. This is known as a *fugue state.*

Hysterical *stupor* is rare and usually only occurs after intense and prolonged stress. Patients become motionless and have to be hand fed. Similar baby-like behaviour, without stupor, occurs in hysterical *puerilism.* Such patients behave as though aged three or four years. Or a hysteric may behave like a dement. During this state of *pseudo-dementia* he will answer questions in a way so absurd as to make it obvious that he knows the real answer i.e. '2 + 2 = 5; a cow has 5 legs; 2 cows have 9 legs.' Often he will claim total amnesia for his past life.

HYSTERIA AND MALINGERING. By definition, hysterical symptoms occur as a result of *unconscious* mechanisms, and bring some gain to the patient. But it is often impossible to say where unconscious mechanisms end and conscious deception or *malingering* begins. When the gain is very great malingering frequently replaces hysteria. Probably, whenever hysterical amnesia lasts for more than a few weeks there is some degree of malingering.

Doctors are sometimes called upon to distinguish between hysteria and malingering in cases of *compensation or accident neurosis*. Patients with this condition complain of disabling nervous symptoms, headache, dizziness, inability to concentrate, insomnia, loss of libido and so on, after an accidental and often trivial injury. Invariably the patient must believe the accident to have been the fault of someone else, and that he is entitled to financial compensation. Many of these patients have been exceptionally healthy before the accident, and given no signs of hysterical tendencies.

Psychiatric treatment is rarely effective while compensation is pending. After compensation the majority recover spontaneously and return to their old jobs. But in a few cases symptoms continue. It seems probable that cases of compensation neurosis range from 'gross conversion hysteria at one end of the scale to frank malingering at the other'.

Munchausen's syndrome (named after the famous Baron von Munchausen) is a curious condition describing those people who repeatedly seek hospital admission and treatment. They have often had repeated laparotomies. Many have curious clinical signs, unequal pupils, papilloedema like optic discs and so on which, together with their complaints, lead to their admission. These patients are sometimes dependent on opiate drugs, are often psychopathic personalities, and very rarely accept psychiatric help.

In conditions such as *dermatitis artefacta*, the patient is aware of what he is doing from the start. Patients may mutilate their faces and bodies in a horrible and seemingly compulsive manner. One woman, over the course of ten years, gradually lost an arm by dipping it in phenol and causing gangrene.

CAUSES. Hysterical symptoms are the result of *dissociation*. A physical or mental 'function', or part of it, separates from personality and consciousness and operates autonomously and unconsciously.

Hysterical reactions can occur in many people under very severe and prolonged stress. But the majority of hysterical disorders seen today occur after relatively minor stress. The nervous systems of these patients are unable to tolerate much tension and *dissociation* occurs readily.

Genetic and early environmental factors both play a part. Hysteria usually occurs in a characteristic type of personality, obsessional, anxious and psychosexually immature. Patients with gross symptoms are likely to be of below average intelligence, and are peculiarly suggestible in a roundabout way. In terms of Eysenck's personality scale, hysterics show extroversion and neuroticism. Many symptoms are the result of suggestion. Aphonia develops after laryngitis, paralysis follows a mild attack of poliomyelitis, amnesia grows out of a blow on the head, aided perhaps by a tactless remark from a doctor or nurse.

Hysteria is particularly liable to occur during an organic illness such as *disseminated sclerosis* or *cerebral tumour*. Hysterical reactions are also liable to be released by *depressive illnesses*. Severe loss of weight, such as occurs in *anorexia nervosa*, may also bring out hysterical tendencies.

Diagnosis. This must always be based on positive as well as negative findings. There should be positive evidence of immature personality, of past hysterical episodes, of emotional conflict and gain. *Hysteria occurring for the first time in middle age, in the absence of organic or depressive illness, is rare.*

TREATMENT. It is usually fairly easy to uncover conflicts and gains under-lying hysterical symptoms. Sympathetic discussion, intravenous barbit-urates or hypnosis may be employed. Hysterical symptoms then disappear, and are usually replaced by those of anxiety.

However, in order to prevent relapse it is then essential to help the patient to deal with his problems. This is best achieved through psycho-therapy, sometimes combined with minor tranquillizers. Physical factors, like loss of weight, must also be treated.

OBSESSIONAL AND COMPULSIVE NEUROSIS

DEFINITION. An obsession is a thought, image, feeling, impulse, or move-ment which an individual feels compelled to carry out, usually repetitively, in spite of a strong urge to resist. He recognizes that this thought or behaviour is absurd and undesirable, but he cannot dispel it.

Obsessions must be distinguished from (1) *delusions,* where the idea or impulse is accepted as reasonable and is not resisted, and (2) *over-valued ideas,* like superstitions, which fall midway between the two. Obsessional compulsive states have much in common, and often co-exist with phobias. Thus an obsession that a woman might kill her child resulted in her phobically avoiding knives.

INCIDENCE. *Obsessional behaviour* is common in children, and again in old age as personality becomes less adaptable. *Obsessional neurosis* occurs most frequently in late adolescence and early adulthood. Single and trans-itory obsessions occur from time to time in many people. These include catchy tunes, absurd phrases, impulses to jump off high places or in front of approaching trains.

SYMPTOMS. Symptoms can be described under three headings:

1. *Obsessional thoughts.* These are usually of an unpleasant nature. Blasphemous, aggressive or sexual thoughts continuously run through the mind. Fears concerning dirt, germs, and venereal disease may arise in response to guilt aroused by masturbation or some sexual incident. These sometimes become linked to religious obsessions and lead to every action being analysed for fear it be a mortal sin.

Patients frequently ruminate on unanswerable problems, such as 'Why are we here?'; 'Is there a God?'; 'Am I really alive?' Students feel compelled to check back to original sources for every statement, and to write an essay or read a chapter of a book may take weeks. Clerks have to check and recheck their work and are only able to keep up to date by working late into the night. Patients may become so slow and indecisive as a result of endless consideration of the pros and cons of every action, that everyday life comes to a halt. This is known as *folie de doubte*.

2. *Impulses*. Obsessional impulses are frequently of an aggressive or suicidal nature. A patient feels an impulse to strangle her child, knife her husband, shout obscene words in church, or misbehave in public. Such feelings, which are often directed against those whom patients love most, cause intense anxiety and distress. However, it is excessively rare for patients to give way to such impulses (in the absence of serious depression), and they can usually be safely reassured.

3. *Compulsions*. Compulsions may arise on their own or as a defence against an obsession. For example, an obsessional fear of germs or dirt may lead to compulsive washing rituals. This secondary compulsion is not resisted as much as the obsessional fears of dirt, and tension is not so marked.

Compulsions may be concerned with sexual or destructive obsessions. A girl of twenty was obsessed with the idea that she might become pregnant as a result of seminal fluid being present on anything she touched or sat upon. Before she sat down she wiped the seat seven times, or a multiple of seven. She changed her underclothes seven times a day, and dressed and undressed seven times on each occasion. If interrupted, she had to start all over again.

A man became obsessed with the thought that he might leave a piece of glass in his used milk bottle. This he thought would be overlooked in the dairy and the customer receiving that bottle of milk would die. He therefore washed each bottle in a special way twenty-five times, five times a day.

Both these patients realized that what they were doing was absurd, but were unable to prevent their actions.

Resistance to such compulsions results in increasing tension until eventually they are carried out. This gives a short-lived feeling of dull relief until the compulsion returns again. Many patients be come depressed by their symptoms, and this in turn causes obsessional and compulsive symptoms to increase.

Unreality and depersonalization are quite common symptoms in obsessional neuroses. Symptoms usually begin suddenly and strongly.

MEDICO LEGAL. Although obsessional impulses and thoughts are frequently of an aggressive nature, they rarely result in harm to others. But sometimes sexual offences and cases of arson seem to be compulsive. Possibly the personality of this type of obsessional patient is less rigid than most. Resistance to the compulsion builds up tension to a level at which consciousness becomes clouded, so that fantasy is 'acted out', and the crime is then committed.

CAUSES

1. Heredity and early environmental influences are obviously important, but are difficult to separate. Obsessional parents not only pass on their genes, but are likely to bring up their children in an obsessional way. Over three-quarters of the patients who develop obsessional neuroses

show, prior to the onset of symptoms, obsessional personality features. And over a third of the parents of these patients have had obsessional, anxiety or depressive illnesses.

2. An obsessional personality who becomes depressed is likely to develop obsessional symptoms. The presence of obsessional symptoms in depressive illness militates against suicide.

3. Schizophrenia may be ushered in by what appears at first to be an obsessional neurosis. Usually such obsessions have a bizarre quality and the patient may not be altogether sure of their absurdity. Their presence lessens the risk of serious personality deterioration.

4. Obsessional symptoms may be caused by organic conditions, such as encephalitis lethargica and brain damage.

TREATMENT AND PROGNOSIS. When severe symptoms occur in childhood the outlook is poor. Most obsessional illnesses develop slowly between the ages of fifteen and twenty-five. Many recover spontaneously within six to twelve months and some of these have no further trouble. However symptoms tend to recur, and after each episode the prognosis is less good. Symptoms generally become less troublesome in middle age. About two-thirds of patients seen by psychiatrists improve or recover fully. If symptoms have persisted unabated for more than five years the prognosis becomes poor. Increased responsibility at work or in the home is likely to cause obsessional symptoms to worsen. On the other hand danger and excitement results in improvement, as many patients discovered during the past war.

1. Psychotherapeutic support and help in avoiding or reducing anxiety are valuable, and may be all that is required in mild cases. Analysis and interpretative psychotherapy should be avoided for, in general, these do more harm than good in such cases.

2. Tranquillizing drugs, especially small doses of phenothiazines, are useful in reducing anxiety. Particularly where phobias co-exist, a combination of phenelzine with a tranquillizer is helpful.

3. In recurring obsessional states, and where obsessional symptoms are coloured by depression, anti-depressive therapy with drugs or *electro convulsive therapy* may be effective. But anti-depressive treatment will not help pure obsessional states.

4. Behaviour therapy, particularly flooding, modelling (imitation learning), or methods which prevent a patient from carrying out his compulsive acts (atropetic therapy) provide the most promising types of treatment available.

5. Severe long-standing obsessional states, causing patients to be crippled by their symptoms, may be greatly improved by prefrontal leucotomy.

SEXUAL ABNORMALITIES AND PROBLEMS

Sexual development has already been described on p. 57. Although the foundations of sex are laid down in utero, and our adult sexual drive and performance are dependent upon and influenced by hormonal factors, much of our sexual behaviour is learnt in the early years of childhood; we learn that we are male or female. Most of us are heterosexual, that is we are mainly attracted to members of the opposite sex. But about 4 per cent of both sexes are homosexual and are attracted wholly or mainly to members of the same sex. A much higher proportion indulge in occasional homosexual behaviour, although they are basically heterosexual.

Some people are attracted strongly to objects other than human beings. These people are known as *fetishists*, and the object of their sexual desire a *fetish*. Nearly all fetishists are male. Common fetishes are female clothing, especially underwear, shoes, hair, rubber and plastic sheets, silk and fur. Most fetishists are heterosexual. The fetish symbolizes and replaces a woman, and thereby becomes the object of sexual desire and the means by which the fetishist achieves sexual orgasm. A fetishist may be able to have intercourse with a woman and reach a climax, provided he can fantasize his fetish. Thus a *transvestite* wearing his wife's underpants and stockings was able to make love to his wife without difficulty. When she objected and refused to let him dress in her clothing he become impotent.

Fetishists are fearful sexually of women unless 'protected' by their fetish. So also are *exhibitionists*, who are only capable of erection and orgasm when they expose themselves to an unknown frightened woman. Peeping Tom or voyeurs masturbate to orgasm while watching an unknown woman undress. The obscene telephone caller has an orgasm while talking to an unknown female. *Coprophiliacs* achieve sexual gratification through eating faeces or being defaecated on by a woman. *Urophiliacs* derive similar pleasure from urine.

Sadism and *masochism* occur in both sexes, although probably more in the male. The sadist is aroused to orgasm by tying up his partner and subjecting her to 'discipline', i.e. by reprimanding and then beating her. The masochist can only obtain satisfaction through being tortured and beaten. Some degree of sadomasochism is common in the fore play to lovemaking of many couples, biting, hair pulling, and so on, but it is then of secondary, not primary importance. For the masochist and the sadist, sexual pleasure is impossible without bondage and punishment. Occasionally the sadist's sense of reality is totally lost. He becomes carried away by his sadistic needs and seriously harms or even kills his partner.

Transvestites enjoy dressing in female clothing. Many masturbate to orgasm after going through the ritual of dressing up. Others ejaculate spontaneously, excited by the feeling of the clothes. Single articles only may be worn, or the transvestite may make himself up as a female, complete with wig and high heels. Transvestism is a common deviation. Probably about 10 per cent of men derive some pleasure from dressing as a women in reality or fantasy, which accounts of course for the popularity of 'drag' shows. Transvestites are mostly heterosexual. Unlike *transexuals* they do not wish to become, nor do they see themselves as, women. Rather, female clothing is their fetish.

Transexualism is the desire to change sex, for a man to become a woman or vice versa. The transexual's sexual drive is usually low. Some of them undergo surgery. Many of them take hormones and dress and live as members of the opposite sex.

Our sexual inclinations and needs are learnt at an early age, probably by three. Fetishists are aware of the pleasure and attraction of their fetish object from early years, although the compulsive sexual need for it only develops strongly at puberty. Transexuals have longed to change their sex since childhood or early puberty. The majority of people with sexual deviations accept and adapt to their needs. Only when the need is of an antisocial nature, and is so strong that it is acted out, does the problem become a medical or legal one.

Treatment of sexual deviations is always difficult. Behaviour therapy offers the most. In serious antisocial cases cyproterone acetate, a drug that neutralizes male sex hormones, can be considered. Castration and psycho-surgery are methods used only in other countries.

IMPOTENCE AND FRIGIDITY. When a man is unable to obtain erection of his penis, or ejaculates so quickly (*premature ejaculation*) that he barely has time to penetrate, he is said to be *impotent*.

Most cases of impotence have psychological causes. Impotence may occur on the first night of the honeymoon, or when husband and wife are reunited after a long separation. In such cases impotence is the result of anxiety. When the man can relax and cease to worry, his sexual potency returns. But sometimes a vicious circle occurs particularly in over-anxious, uncertain young men who regard each attempt at intercourse as a trial. Inevitably they continue to fail.

Sometimes impotence occurs after years of apparently satisfactory sexual relationship. This may reflect a man's growing resentment for his wife. In other instances impotence may be a symptom of depression, or of an organic condition such as diabetes.

Frigidity, and *dyspareunia*, which is the female equivalent of impotence, is also largely the result of uncertainty and anxiety. Some women are frigid because they are terrified of pregnancy.

Treatment. From the point of view of treating impotence, it is important to know whether the man is impotent only with one or all women. It is not uncommon to find that during pre-marital intercourse a couple had a good sexual relationship, and only after marriage or just before the wedding did impotence or frigidity develop. Such sexual disturbances reflect neurotic conflicts in one or both partners. Fantasies which can exist with a mistress or prostitute may not be possible with a wife. At marriage a wife succeeds, and in a sense displaces, her husband's mother. So also a husband steps into the shoes of his wife's father. Unresolved conflicts and ties with parent figures need to be explored before treatment can be decided upon.

Sometimes sexual difficulties are due to a mixture of ignorance and anxiety. These can be simply corrected by a sensible, reassuring discussion with the couple. Resentments between partners may need to be brought out. It is important to impress upon the couple that the trouble lies not so much in either partner as in the nature of their sexual relationship. A good sexual relationship is based on communication and trust. The man who can only enjoy sex with a call girl and never with his wife, the woman who is unable to feel sexual desire for any man she loves, is unlikely to develop a satisfying marriage.

Tranquillizers before intercourse may help to reduce anxiety. Anti-depressants are logical if impotence is due to depression, but it must be remembered that impotence is sometimes a side effect of such drugs. Behaviour therapy is useful. Fantasies need to be explored, and pornographic literature or 'shows' are sometimes valuable for releasing a couple's mutual inhibitions. *Marital group therapy* is sometimes helpful.

12

PAIN AND PSYCHOSOMATIC DISORDERS

Emotional factors enter into almost every patient's illness. Every patient feels some anxiety about himself when he first attends hospital. He may consequently exaggerate or minimize his symptoms according to his personality. In other instances, emotional factors may produce disturbance of function and physical symptoms when no organic disease exists. Between a third and a quarter of patients attending general practice surgeries have no detectable organic disease to account for their symptoms.

The term psychosomatic, then, in its widest sense, can be applied to almost every medical or surgical condition. But such a wide concept reduces the usefulness of the term. It is better, therefore, to limit the use of the term to the following three groups:

1. Patients who have somatic symptoms but no evidence of organic disease.

2. Patients whose symptoms can be brought on or exacerbated by emotional factors, but where organic changes are found, e.g. ulcerative colitis.

3. Patients with illnesses which are intimately related to disturbances of the autonomic system, and where emotional factors often play a part, e.g. asthma, migraine.

Psychosomatic illnesses usually involve those parts of the body which are composed of smooth muscle and glandular structures, controlled by the autonomic and endocrine systems. A vicious circle is present in many psychosomatic states, perpetuating symptoms even when the causative factors no longer exist. Many of the illnesses respond to simple reassurance and explanation that no organic disease exists. Many patients, with say asthma or peptic ulcer, will respond when removed from their environment, for instance on coming into hospital. However, many of them relapse on returning home.

Some people have tried to show that specific types of personality develop particular psychosomatic illnesses. This is not so, although it is certainly true that patients with psychosomatic illnesses tend to have obsessive personalities and to bottle up their feelings. It is likely however that chronic illness itself will bring about personality changes. Other people have tried unsuccessfully to show that a psychosomatic illness

121

symbolizes, or is an expression of, a particular kind of conflict. While it is true that some people who suffer from migraine do persistently suppress feelings of resentment and hostility, many do not, and other factors must be concerned.

It is not always easy to separate psychological from other causal factors. Sometimes the first attack of asthma or colitis may have been due to an infection, or a substance to which the patient is allergic. This 'sensitizes' him and subsequently a variety of factors, including psychological, can bring about the same reaction.

Advantages may accrue from a patient's physical symptoms. Pain always evokes a sympathetic response from nurses and doctors, and from the patient's relatives and friends. A patient's reactions to discomfort are sometimes exaggerated or prolonged in order to avoid an unpleasant or feared situation. For instance, a child who dislikes school or fears to leave his mother may exaggerate the pain of his sprained ankle, or the symptoms of a mild upper respiratory tract infection.

Pain is used by some patients as a means of communication, an appeal for love and sympathy, an expression of resentment, an excuse for a sense of failure and impotence. We are still remarkably ignorant about the mechanism of pain. Emotional attitudes and past experiences play an important part in the way a patient feels and reacts to pain. A soldier may not even notice a severe wound received in the heat of battle. But at another time a minor wound evokes severe pain. Some patients over-react when a particular part of their body is damaged. And sometimes an injury which should be painful produces pleasurable sensations. This is most obvious in sadomasochism. Personality plays a part in pain reaction. Introverts have a lower threshold for pain than extraverts, although the latter tend to complain more readily. Depressed patients frequently express their misery solely through complaints of pain; the most common sites are head, abdomen, chest, limbs and face, in that order.

EXAMPLES OF PSYCHOSOMATIC STATES AFFECTING DIFFERENT SYSTEMS

THE CARDIOVASCULAR SYSTEM. Fear and anxiety cause *tachycardia* and palpitations. When associated with breathlessness, discomfort over the heart, fear of dying, and sweating this is known as *effort syndrome* or *cardiac neurosis*. The secondary anxiety provoked by these symptoms sometimes creates a state of panic and collapse. Occasionally parasympathetic activity predominates. When a slow pulse coincides with a low blood pressure fainting is likely. In anorexia nervosa the pulse may slow to as low as 40 beats a minute.

The role of emotion in causing *essential hypertension* is uncertain. But that emotion can raise blood pressure temporarily, particularly systolic, is not disputed. Anxiety and depression probably play some part in cases of coronary thrombosis. Bereavement is certainly followed by an increased incidence of heart attacks.

THE SKIN. Fear produces pallor, sham produces blushing. Chronic anxiety is often associated with a greasy sweaty skin. Acne and infection are then more likely to develop.

Emotional factors play a part in eczema, although the importance of this varies from patient to patient. If emotional factors are not present, then psychotherapeutic treatment may increase rather than diminish the eczema.

Pruritus is common in many skin conditions. Scratching may become compulsive and then perpetuate the skin trouble.

THE RESPIRATORY SYSTEM. *Asthma, hay fever, vasomotor-rhinitis* are reactions to a mixture of allergic, constitutional and psychological factors. A full-blown asthmatic attack is terrifying both to the patient and his relatives. This may lead the mother of an asthmatic child to adopt an over-protective attitude to the child. The child will feel resentful and angry, and inhibition of his feelings may make matters worse. It is important to recognize that many factors are involved in asthma (and many other psychosomatic states), and that their effects summate. Every case of asthma has an immunological basis. Although emotional factors may be obvious these are not necessarily the prime cause.

Over-breathing occurs in anxiety states and in agitated depression. If this is prolonged alkalosis and tetany develop.

THE GASTRO-INTESTINAL TRACT. About 10 per cent of patients in general and hospital practice present with gastro-intestinal symptoms. Yet only about half have any diagnosable organic cause. Emotions affect the mucous membranes of the gastro-intestinal tract in different ways. The best known study is of Tom, a boy who was unable to swallow and had an artificial opening made into his stomach through the abdomen. Fear caused the gastric mucosa to become congested and engorged, so that it bled when touched. Depression caused the mucosa to become pale, and decreased gastric motility and secretion.

Vomiting is a common reaction to emotional upsets and tensions. It may also be present in anorexia nervosa and depression. A few people vomit regularly, usually in the morning, without any other symptoms. In such cases vomiting seems to have become a habit following a specific gastric or psychological upset.

The *irritable bowel syndrome* (spastic colitis) is a common recurring condition of abdominal pain and/or diarrhoea, sometimes interspersed with constipation. Twice as many women as men are affected. Stress is responsible for most attacks of this syndrome. There is no relation between this and ulcerative colitis.

Ulcerative colitis itself is not caused by psychological factors, although subsequently they may influence the course and management of the illness.

Constipation is a subjective state, with a different meaning for different patients. Nearly a quarter of the population of the U.K. take laxatives at least once a week, the habit having been established in childhood. Obsessional preoccupation over bowel activity, and the need to have at least one 'good' movement a day, increases with age. It is sometimes a major symptom of depression.

THE GENITO-URINARY SYSTEM. *Pre-menstrual tension* is common to many women; nearly 40 per cent of otherwise healthy women report troublesome symptoms before menstruation. Pre-menstrual symptoms consist of irritability, anxiety, headache, palpitations, dizziness, and a bloated sensation of abdomen and breasts. Sleep, eating, and sexual libido may be increased or diminished, and the skin becomes greasy and spotty. During the pre-menstrual period and the start of menstruation, women are more liable than usual to shoplift, fail exams, absent themselves from work, attempt suicide, and be involved in road accidents. The pre-menstrual syndrome extends to all ages after puberty, even beyond the menopause. Women with severe symptoms tend to be neurotic personalities.

Dysmenorrhoea on the other hand is not related either to neuroticism or to the pre-menstrual syndrome, although pain may become a focus for the emotional problems of some women. Dyspareunia and vaginismus are usually due to anxiety and fears of sexual intercourse. Oral contraceptives can cause depression, irritability, decreased libido, and headache. About 6 per cent of women on the pill, particularly one with a high progesterone content, report depression. Changes of libido, up or down, may be due as much to the psychological effects of taking the pill as to hormonal ones.

THE ENDOCRINE SYSTEM. *Amenorrhoea* and *menorrhagia* often occur in response to anxiety and depression. Menstruation stops for a variable time in about 25 per cent of nurses and students when they leave home for the first time. Amenorrhoea occurred in 65 per cent of European women interned in Hong Kong in 1940. *Anorexia nervosa* (see p. 125) a syndrome consisting of amenorrhoea and loss of weight, is primarily due to psychological factors, acting through hypothalamic structures.

Thyrotoxicosis and *diabetes* can follow emotional stress, although other factors must play an important part.

MISCELLANEOUS. *Acute intermittent porphyria* is inherited as an autosomal dominant and occurs mainly in young adults. Abdominal pain and vomiting are common features, but depression and hysteria, and even frank psychosis, may be prominent and result in the condition being mistaken for hysteria. Barbiturates and diazepines should never be given.

Cardiac surgery. Patients often develop confusional states a few days after operation. These clear up spontaneously within a week.

Renal dialysis imposes strains not only on the patient but his family and the nursing staff. Insecurity about the future, threat of death, and most of all the fact that the patient is continually dependent upon his machine, the medical staff, and his family, make it difficult for some patients to adapt well to haemodialysis.

ANOREXIA NERVOSA

DEFINITION. Primary anorexia nervosa is a syndrome which occurs mainly in young women. The central feature is loss of weight, due to the patient's active refusal to eat enough, and amenorrhoea. Secondary signs and symptoms of starvation subsequently become increasingly prominent. Hunger is not necessarily lost, and refusal to eat stems from the patient's irrational fears that if she eats she will lose control of her appetite and become increasingly fat.

SYMPTOMS. Typically, symptoms begin while the girl is working for an important leaving examination or scholarship, or soon after she leaves school. She believes that she is too fat and puts herself on to an increasingly exacting diet. She loses weight steadily and eventually her parents and friends begin to express alarm. The girl herself at this stage may realize that she is too thin, but she is now unable to stop her self-imposed starvation. This behaviour, which occasionally results in death, is compulsive.

Secondary effects from the weight loss occur sooner or later. Hunger decreases and in most cases ceases to be troublesome. Foods other than fruit, vegetables and cheese, on which many of these girls subsist, cause a feeling of sickness and epigastic distension. Downy hair grows on the face and limbs. The extremities become bluish-red and the skin cold and rough. The pulse is sometimes as slow as forty beats a minute, and the systolic blood pressure falls below 100 mm. Oedema occurs during extreme emaciation. It is characteristic of these patients to remain very active and alert. But eventually they become so emaciated and weak that they can barely stand erect. Severe loss of weight may itself bring about psychiatric disturbances and sometimes leads to a mistaken diagnosis of schizophrenia. In some cases amenorrhoea or menstrual irregularities will precede the weight loss. Generally, however, amenorrhoea coincides with the onset or follows the weight loss some months later.

A similar refusal to eat, and severe weight loss, occasionally occurs in young men.

CAUSES. Primary anorexia nervosa appears to be on the increase. It is a disease of an affluent society and occurs only when the availability of food is taken for granted and obesity can also exist. During the 19th and early 20th centuries anorexia nervosa was seen mainly only among the wealthy classes. Today, as affluence spreads downwards, it occurs in all except the poorest class. It is also related to intelligence and education and is more common among the pupils of private and grammar schools. Epidemics of anorexia nervosa break out from time to time, particularly in girls' boarding schools (resembling the outbreaks of mass hysteria seen in past centuries in closed female communities) which continue until the ringleader is removed to hospital.

Numerous factors, genetic, constitutional and environmental, probably contribute to the development of anorexia nervosa. Learning obviously plays a major role. The earlier age of onset of puberty may be important, and account for the increasing number of very young patients seen today. Advertising clearly has an influence. Mothers are urged to overfeed their children, but at puberty the adolescent girl is rapidly persuaded of the desirability of slimness. Most adolescent girls try to diet at some time, whether or not they are overweight, if only to keep in the fashion. Overweight is a vague term but probably only about half the patients who develop anorexia nervosa are plump or overweight before dieting. Adolescent males are nothing like so weight conscious as females, which may be an important reason why females outnumber males by 20 to 1 in this respect.

Food often plays a major role in the families of patients. Love and affection are symbolized by food, and eating becomes virtually the only means of a patient communicating and expressing her feelings. Her attitude towards her parents is an ambivalent one, both rejecting by her refusal to eat, at the same time attention seeking. Anorexia nervosa almost invariably leads to open conflict between the patient and her family, and brings family tensions as a whole to the surface.

The build up of aggressive and sexual needs at puberty causes anxiety, particularly if the adolescent lacks a secure background. At 11 or 12 symptoms of anorexia nervosa develop mainly in response to a patient's fear of her growing aggressive urges and to separation anxiety, which are likely to be increased by parental depression. Many of these patients have been model children, well behaved, compliant, clean, tidy, polite and successful at school. They start to become more outgoing and forceful, when some rebuff occurs and arouses their anxiety. An illness or death within the family suddenly causes a patient to become aware and fearful of the consequences of her emerging emotions. Desire for self control, for protection, becomes overwhelming, and achieves rapid satisfaction through dieting.

After puberty, psychosexual conflicts become increasingly important. Most patients are sexually immature and naive, often because of family attitudes. Some scandal may occur at school, a school friend be forced to leave, and the patient's fantasies are aroused, increasing her fears of her own sexuality. In many patients the apparent precipitating cause is often trivial, frequently a G.C.E. examination; fear of failure, usually unrealistic, arouses fear of rejection, loss of parental affection, and builds up into a vicious circle.

Occasionally anorexia nervosa develops just before or after marriage. The prognosis for such a case is not good, because the husband steps directly into the parental boots. Sexual intercourse is only infrequent or absent. Occasionally the diagnosis of anorexia nervosa is confused by the patient taking a contraceptive pill, which delays the onset of amenorrhoea.

DIFFERENTIAL DIAGNOSIS. Loss of weight due to refusal to eat or excessive vomiting can occur in a number of psychiatric conditions. Severe depression is associated with anorexia and often amenorrhoea. A schizophrenic may refuse to eat because of delusional ideas about being poisoned.

Anorexia, loss of weight and menstrual irregularities commonly result from anxiety, particularly of a psychosexual nature, in vulnerable young women. Organic conditions must be excluded, such as thyrotoxicosis, Crohn's disease and pituitary or hypothalamic lesions. It is usually not difficult to exclude these, and any signs of anaemia or vitamin deficiencies should immediately raise doubts about a diagnosis of primary anorexia nervosa.

PROGNOSIS. It is important to know the natural course of anorexia nervosa. The majority of patients improve spontaneously within 6 months to 3 years. As eating inhibitions begin to relax, compulsive over-eating may occur. This is usually short-lived but can persist for years and cause obesity. Depression of mood follows over-eating, which is most often in secret at night. Such a patient sometimes compulsively swallows large quantities of hypnotics and tranquillizers early in the evening in an attempt to stop overeating. This is rarely a true suicidal attempt. Compulsive stealing may also occur at this time, usually of trivial objects. That there is a relationship between such stealing and sexuality is suggested by the fact that stealing stops when sexual inhibitions lift. Menstruation follows a variable time after recovery of a reasonable weight. Rarely menstruation does not return. Patients who have recovered are able to marry and become pregnant without difficulty. Pregnancy and delivery are generally uncomplicated and the birth weights of their babies are within normal range. Some patients remain vulnerable personalities, always mildly obsessed about eating and weight, prone to phobic anxiety, hypochondriasis and reactive depression. Chronic states of anorexia nervosa are uncommon, but are very intractable and potentially dangerous. Psychiatrists tend to see mainly patients with severe or longstanding anorexia nervosa, although general practitioners are now liable to refer them much earlier than before. In the past, about 15 per cent of patients with severe anorexia nervosa died as a result of weight loss, or indirectly from contracting other diseases such as pulmonary tuberculosis. Nowadays this is unlikely.

TREATMENT. Proper treatment must depend on thoroughly understanding a patient's fears, secondary gains and family background. If a patient has lost much weight she will nearly always require treatment in hospital, away from her family. In some cases this may be lifesaving. Nurses should appreciate that the patient is terrified of eating and will resort to any means to avoid it.

In hospital the quickest way of restoring weight is by confining the patient to bed and giving her chlorpromazine, if necessary combined with modified insulin. The starting dose is around 150 mg a day, steadily increasing to 1000 mg a day or even more if necessary. An anti-Parkinsonian drug needs to be given to prevent dystonic reactions. The function of chlorpromazine is to reduce the patient's anxiety, to lessen her resistance to eating, and to prevent her disposing of food. Whether it has a specific therapeutic effect on the hypothalamus is debatable. It is advisable to give light, frequent meals at first, increasing the total calories intake from 1500 to 4000 or 5000 calories a day. A firm but kindly, understanding attitude towards the patient is important. She is given weight targets and when she attains these she is rewarded by some concession; allowed visitors, allowed up to the toilet and so on. Antidepressant drugs are sometimes helpful after weight has been regained.

Psychotherapy has an important part to play but in a supportive, not interpretive sense. The therapist, to succeed, must become a parent substitute, supporting, trusted and to some extent idealized. Some measure of family therapy is also important, since anorexia nervosa is always a family problem. Weekly family group meetings, in addition to seeing the patient individually, may be valuable in relapsing young patients.

Chronic relapsing anorexia nervosa may be suitable for modified prefrontal leucotomy. Patients carefully selected have done extremely well following operation. Menstruation has returned, weight has stabilized at a good level and the patient is able to lead an independent working life and sometimes marry.

Young nurses often have considerable emotional problems and difficulties in treating anorexia nervosa, particularly if they identify with the patient's problems. It is not unknown for a nurse to collude with a patient in disposing of her food. Conversely, a nurse may find it difficult not to lose her temper with a patient refusing to eat.

13

AFFECTIVE DISORDERS

DEPRESSIVE ILLNESS

DEFINITION. A feeling of sadness, despair or inexplicable disinterest, is probably experienced by most people at some time. Characteristically it follows the loss or abandonment of some much wanted ambition or object. When personal loss is severe sadness deepens and becomes grief. The mourner for a time becomes preoccupied by painful memories and thoughts. Gradually these fade and life resumes its former course.

But sometimes sadness and grief are prolonged or exaggerated beyond what seems reasonable. Depression ceases to be merely a symptom and becomes an illness, involving widespread depression of mental and physical functions. The patient becomes slow and indecisive, increasingly incapable of coping with his everyday problems. Physical symptoms often predominate, particularly in milder depressions, not only because bodily functions are upset but because depression lowers the appreciation of and tolerance for bodily discomfort.

Depression is twice as common in women as in men. The incidence of depression in the U.K. is rising, to judge by first admission rates to psychiatric hospitals and units. The prevalence increases with age and reaches a peak in late middle age. About 1 in 10 of the population is liable to develop a depressive illness at some stage in his life.

CLASSIFICATION OF DEPRESSION. The term *endogenous* or *psychotic* depression implies that genetic and constitutional factors are more important than external stresses as causes. *Reactive* or *neurotic* or *psychogenic* depression suggests that external pressures and neurotic personality features play the major role. Psychiatrists differ in the way they classify depressive illness. Some regard depression as a continuum, stretching uniformly from psychotic to neurotic depression, to be understood mainly in psychological terms. Others see depression as a mixture of separate disorders, each with their own aetiology, prognosis and treatment. They separate endogenous depression clearly from neurotic depression.

Endogenous depression comprises *manic* depression, or bipolar affective disorder, and involutional melancholia. Not everyone agrees that involutional melancholia, characterized by agitation and hypochondriasis, is a separate entity, and a number of clinical and genetic studies suggest that it does not differ from other psychotic depressions. Since the advent of effective modern treatments these disagreements are more of academic than practical importance.

SYMPTOMS. Symptoms of depression are protean. Depression is both easy and difficult to diagnose, for there are not only psychological symptoms but physical as well, However, severe depression is usually unmistakable. The patient looks miserable and pessimism colours his outlook. He is indecisive, hopeless, and continually blaming himself for past peccadillos or imaginary failures. He sees only ruin and disgrace ahead. He may show marked retardation with little spontaneous movement or talk. He may be extremely *agitated*, continually pacing the floor, wringing his hands or clasping his head. Sometimes he shows both *retardation* and *agitation*. His sleep is nearly always disturbed and typically he wakes in the early hours, when depression tends to be at its worst. In the beginning the depression may lighten as the day lengthens, but later there is no lift whatever. There is usually profound anorexia and loss of weight. Constipation is a common complaint and there may be delusional ideas of being blocked or rotting internally, mixed with hypochondriacal preoccupation. Sexual interest is lost and menstruation may cease. There may be depersonalization and unreality feelings.

Milder depressions are less typical and present in a variety of ways. Occasionally the patient smiles and jokes about his symptoms, although underneath he may be suicidal. Often he complains merely of fatigue and irritability, of waking tired and unrefreshed, or of no longer being able to cope with his work.

Many patients complaining of physical symptoms for which no organic cause can be found are suffering from a *masked depression*. Abdominal pain and nausea are common symptoms which may lead to prolonged investigations. Careful questioning will show that the patient is depressed, that the pain is really an unpleasant churning sensation in the epigastrium and is at its worst on wakening. Headaches can be severe and take the form of a tight band around or a heavy pressure on the head. Pain in the back is not infrequent, and many a slipped disc hides a depression. Cardiovascular symptoms are sometimes attributed to 'blood pressure' and treatment with antihypertensive drugs may make matters worse. Palpitations, dizziness and flushings lead to increasing anxiety and may, in women, be attributed to 'the change'. Loss of sexual potency and interest are less likely to be regarded as organic, but are sometimes dismissed as due to middle age. This may sometimes lead to marital troubles, for instance, when a wife attributes her husband's failures to infidelity.

Some depressions present as anxiety states and the underlying depression may easily be overlooked. Phobias connected with travelling, harming people, of madness or of some fatal disease are common. When occurring suddenly in middle life without apparent cause, they should always bring depression to mind. Many of the differences in depressive symptoms are related to individual differences in personality. For instance, when very obsessional people become depressed they may develop severe ruminations or compulsions. One woman who has had recurring bouts of depression since her husband died is compelled during an attack always to rent an expensive flat, far beyond her means, although she has a comfortable home of her own. Another patient is forced to steal goods from display counters and subsequently to return them. Such behaviour is distressing to the patient but she seems unable to resist when depressed. In others psychopathic behaviour is released. A faithful spouse may suddenly go off the rails, become promiscuous and leave his family, or start to drink excessively. Equally suddenly the depression may lift and the psychopathy disappear. Unless it is realized that a medical rather than a moral judgement is needed, a previously happy home may be broken.

There is invariably some loss of insight in depression and the patient's explanation of his illness should always be suspect until confirmed. He may blame an unsatisfactory job, home or marriage for his depression, whereas the reverse may be the case. It is essential to prevent the patient from doing anything he may later regret. Any suggestion that he should change his job or leave his wife should be firmly opposed until he has fully recovered. Only then is he capable of making responsible decisions.

Depression may occur at any age. Some authorities deny that it occurs in children, but this seems to be a quibble rather than a fact, and a condition resembling depression is clearly seen in some children. Moodiness in adolescence is normal, but a full-blown depression can also occur, although this may herald a schizophrenic illness. The incidence of depressive illness increases steadily with age until the senium. Recent work has shown how frequently potentially recoverable depressions occur in old age and how important it is to distinguish them from senile dementia whose prognosis is hopeless.

CLINICAL TYPES OF DEPRESSION

Specific clinical types of depressive illness are described, although in practice it may be difficult to distinguish one clearly from another.

1. *Reactive or Neurotic Depression.* Symptoms of *anxiety* colour those of depression. The depression is not generally very deeply rooted and may be temporarily lifted by pleasant company or a change of surroundings. Symptoms tend to be at their worst at the end of the day or when the patient is alone. Symptoms of anxiety and tension have often been present for many months, even years, before the onset of depression. Suicidal feelings are common but suicide itself is rare, although self-poisoning gestures may occur.

2. *Endogenous depression*

(a) *Manic depression (bipolar).* Kraepelin (1896) was the first to link mania and depression. He pointed out the good prognosis for spontaneous recovery, but also the tendency for recurrence. Manic depression can start at any age, but the first attack is usually between twenty and thirty-five years, and is usually depressive in nature. Many patients never have an attack of mania. In others mania alternates with depression or occurs intermittently. Only relatively few patients have attacks of mania alone.

Patients with manic depression tend to have an endomorphic/mesomorphic type of body build, and to have cyclothymic extroverted personalities. Many are successful in their work, and the onset of depression with loss of drive and zest, unreasonable anxiety and pessimism creates considerable problems. Retardation is often prominent. Delusions of guilt and unworthiness may develop into delusions of persecution. Anorexia, weight loss and insomnia are marked. Physical changes are sometimes striking: the skin becomes pale, bouts of sweating occur, hair lacks lustre, boils and skin infections develop, eyelids droop and muscle tone diminishes. Depressive attacks last from a few days or weeks to years. The average time is between 6 to 18 months, but each patient tends to follow his own characteristic pattern. Attacks often develop suddenly with little or no prodromal warning signs, and may lift as dramatically. Attacks sometime occur at the same time each year, particularly spring and autumn, several times a year, intermittently at long intervals, or once only. When manic depression attacks occur after the age of fifty there is a high risk of recurrence.

Recovery from depression is usually followed by an upsurge of energy and enhanced sense of enjoyment. This can be looked upon as normal, and gradually disappears. But in some patients mania or hypomania (a mild form of mania) develop.

(b) *Unipolar depression.* This describes recurrent attacks of depression without mania. There is some genetic evidence that unipolar differs from bipolar affective illness, but it is usually impossible to rule out the possibility of a manic episode in the future.

(c) *Involutional melancholia.* This type of depression, beginning in middle age, is characterized by agitation rather than retardation (although in practice a mixture of both is usually present), hypochondriasis and paranoid delusions. If untreated, it has a poor prognosis. In fact there is considerable doubt as to whether involutional depression is a separate entity. In any case the prognostic significance of the diagnosis is lost since patients respond well to ECT and antidepressant drugs.

(d) *Depression in childhood.* See p. 162.

AETIOLOGY

1. Genetic factors are probably important. In manic depression a dominant gene with incomplete penetrance has been postulated. The concordance rates for identical and non-identical twins is 68 per cent and 23 per cent respectively, which suggests a strong genetic influence. The risk of first-degree relatives of a patient developing manic depression is considerably greater than in the general population, approaching 15 per cent.

A clear relationship exists between age of onset at first attack and genetic factors. Patients who develop depression for the first time after 50, and even more after the age of 65, are much less likely to possess a positive family history of affective disorder than young patients. In older patients therefore physical illness and external stresses are perhaps of greater causal importance.

2. Biochemical changes are known to be associated with depression and mania, although these may be the result rather than the cause of the attack.

The monoamine theory of depression is based on findings that noradrenaline and 5-hydroxytryptamine (5HT), which are both neurotransmitters in the brain (see p. 72), are depleted in depression and increased in mania. The evidence for this comes from (a) animal studies, (b) changes in the concentration of these substances in the CSF during affective disorders, (c) depleted amounts of monoamines in the brains of people who have committed suicide, and (d) evidence from the use of drugs in man, which either increase or deplete brain amines.

Output from the adrenal glands is increased in both depression and mania, probably a stress effect secondary to the disorder itself.

3. Early childhood experiences, both psychological and physical, are important and may, by a conditioning process, invest the factor precipitating the illness with its emotional significance. Thus the loss of a parent in early childhood predisposes that person to depression in later life following a 'loss'.

4. Cultural influences affect both the incidence and the symptomatology of depressive illness. It is claimed that affective disorders are most common among 'people who have a high degree of social cohesion and are group centred'. Depression is inversely related to the open expression of aggression. Depressive illness and suicide rates invariably drop during times of war and during riots (see under Suicide, p. 136).

Depression seems to be comparatively uncommon in primitive societies, and when it does occur tends to be characterized by hypochondriacal and paranoid symptoms. Self-blame and a sense of guilt, which occur so frequently in our culture, are almost never seen and suicide is rare. In our society depression is thought to be increasing, particularly in older patients, although whether the increase is real or only apparent is hard to say.

A sense of isolation often results in depression. Old people living on their own, hampered perhaps by deafness or bad eyesight, are prone to become depressed. Lonely single people are more likely to kill themselves than those living with their families, as a recent London survey has shown. But even families are not immune from isolation and depression. A survey of a new estate has shown that the incidence of neurotic illness is about 50 per cent higher than the average for the whole country, 'neurotic reactive depression in women' predominating. The conclusion from this survey was that each family 'kept itself to itself', producing loneliness and social isolation that led to psychiatric symptoms.

Depression often occurs after a virus infection such as influenza, infective hepatitis, glandular fever, after operations, particularly hysterectomy, the puerperium and with organic states. Drugs such as cortisone or reserpine may also cause severe depression. It has been estimated that about 10 per cent of patients treated for hypertension with reserpine develop depression. Weight loss can also be a precipitating factor and too-enthusiastic slimmers are often seen in psychiatric clinics. Psychological factors have already been mentioned and it is apparent that no single factor is sufficient to explain the occurrence of depression.

TREATMENT. When discussing the value of treatment in affective disorders, it is always as well to remember that spontaneous recovery is virtually the rule.

The breakdown of any individual is probably the result, ultimately, of some physical or chemical dysfunction in the nervous system. The fundamental causes are not known, but it seems likely that neurotransmitter substances or enzymes in the brain, particularly the monoamines, play some part in the regulation of mood and are disturbed in affective disorders. Antidepressant drugs are believed to exert their therapeutic effect by raising the concentration of these substances.

Antidepressant drugs are not general euphoriants. They fall into two main groups, and have been in clinical use since about 1957. The *tricyclic antidepressants* which include imipramine and amitriptyline, are the more widely used, and are particularly useful in the endogenous type of depressive illness. The *monoamine oxidase inhibitors* (MAOI), iproniazid, phenelzine, tranylcypromine, are more useful in reactive forms of depression, particularly when associated with features of phobic anxieties. However, it is impossible to be too didactic about the indications for each, and it is often a question of trial and error. In most cases it is best to begin treatment with a tricyclic antidepressant since this is safer than a MAOI, and it is easier to change quickly to a MAOI than vice versa if the patient fails to respond. With both groups of antidepressants there is a delay of up to a fortnight, usually 5–10 days, before therapeutic effects begin to show, while side effects appear almost immediately. It is important to tell the patient about this. The antidepressant drugs are not curative. They suppress symptoms and allow a patient to cope and if necessary sort out his life problems until spontaneous remission occurs. They must be continued therefore for years if necessary. Stopping the drug too soon brings on relapse. (For details of dosage, side and toxic effects, etc., see p. 184).

Amphetamines are now rarely used except for a few middle-aged neurotic depressives who have been maintained for years on 5–10 mg a day. The euphoric effects tend to be transitory and are sometimes followed by an increased sense of depression. There is also a danger that the patient may become dependent on the drug.

Tranquillizers, either diazepine derivatives or small doses of a phenothiazine such as trifluoperazine or perphenazine, are often combined with an antidepressant if anxiety or agitation are severe. The tranquillizers have no specific antidepressant action but many anxious patients undoubtedly feel more cheerful when their anxiety is relieved. Older patients in particular, with symptoms of mild anxiety and depression respond to a tranquillizer alone.

L-tryptaphon (*Optimax*), which is the precursor of 5HT, is claimed to relieve depression and to have few side effects. It does potentiate the action of the MAOI group, but alone or with the tricyclic antidepressants seems to have little effect.

Mania and hypomania require treatment with chlorpromazine and/or haloperidol. Up to 1000 mg a day of chlorpromazine and 60 mg of haloperidol may be needed in acute mania. If the patient is unco-operative, intramuscular or intravenous injections are necessary. 20–30 mg of haloperidol intravenously two or three times a day usually controls mania within a few days. Subsequently lithium carbonate should be considered if there is a history of recurrent attacks of mania and depression.

Electro-convulsive therapy (*ECT*) is still the most effective treatment for depression and should be given at once if there is a serious risk of suicide. It should never be withheld for too long when a patient fails to respond fully to antidepressant drug therapy. ECT and drugs can be combined with safety. ECT is still occasionally used for the treatment of mania. It must then be given much more frequently, once or twice a day, until there is improvement, usually within a few days.

Psychotherapy and help in solving emotional problems are often required but it is best to avoid comments and interpretations, or even advice, until depression has clearly begun to lift. Psychotherapy done too early or clumsily is liable to increase a depressed patient's sense of guilt and self-blame, and precipitate a suicide attempt. However, psychotherapy, individual or group, is often invaluable for patients with neurotic forms of depression.

NURSING CARE. Nursing care involves attention to all the physical symptoms which may accompany a depressive illness. Psychological care is aimed at increasing a patient's feeling of worth and self confidence, but it is not easy to convince a depressed patient that life is still worth living. The nurse should encourage the patient to participate in ward activities and entertainments, but should not force him before he is ready. He should not, on the other hand, be allowed to isolate himself completely.

If the patient expresses suicidal ideas the nurse must be especially vigilant. She must discreetly observe the patient at all times and ensure that he does not have access to any means of suicide, such as drugs, sharp instruments and so on.

MANIA AND HYPOMANIA

DEFINITION. *Mania* is the opposite of depression. The patient is elated, optimistic and extremely quick, both mentally and physically. In his conversation he shows *flight of ideas*, and the topic is continually changed. But the changes are always understandable and connected to one another, unlike the disconnected talk of a schizophrenic. The manic patient is liable to be lacking in tact, disinhibited and often very amusing. He is always on the go, is distractful and easily irritated. Grandiose schemes are started only to be dropped for something even greater. There is generally little time for food or sleep, but sometimes he pursues women and spends money recklessly. Judgement is faulty and he may run foul of the law.

Extreme states of mania result in patients becoming unmanageable outside hospital. Delusions, hallucinations, both visual and auditory, and aggressive excitement may be prominent. The milder forms, known as *hypomania*, merge imperceptibly with normal states of elation.

NURSING CARE.   Manic patients should be nursed in quiet, non-stimulating surroundings; ideally in a single room, under sedation. Full nursing care is necessary, with special attention given to an adequate fluid intake, diet and personal cleanliness.

The nurse should be tactful in her dealings with the manic patient, who may laugh with her at one moment but be highly irritable the next. These patients are usually very interfering and can cause havoc in a peaceful ward. When the patient is up and about, it is usually best to provide him with some occupation. It is useless, however, to expect him to continue with one activity for any length of time.

SUICIDE

The official suicide rate in England and Wales has declined over the last 10 years from 120 to 80 per million. Men still outnumber women by 2 to 1 but the female proportion is increasing, particularly in elderly women. There is disagreement about how reliable these official figures are. The majority of people who kill themselves, probably over 90 per cent, are psychiatrically disturbed, depressive illness being the most common. A high proportion, just before their death, have gone to their G.P. but failed to obtain help. Many have made one or more abortive attempts before the final act. In other words, suicide rarely comes out of the blue but is preceded by warning signs. Late middle age is when suicide is most likely. Alcoholism increases the risk.

Many factors contribute to suicide. It was Durkheim who pointed out the relationship between suicide and the way in which a person is integrated in his society and controlled by its norms and values, especially those concerning death and suicide. Those who are and feel socially isolated are more prone to suicide. Marriage and children, active religion, a settled home, all lessen the risk of suicide. The suicide rate is highest among the single, divorced and separated, among those who emigrate or move to an unfamiliar area, and is greater in urban than in rural areas. Sudden stress, particularly bereavement, financial worry, and legal disputes may prove the last straw for the middle-aged depressive already near breaking point. Drugs are the common method of suicide, usually obtained from a doctor. In the past gassing was frequently used, but natural gas has removed that possibility. Depressives sometimes employ particularly unpleasant methods; throat cutting, swallowing corrosive liquids, hanging, drowning, jumping in front of a train. Suicide nearly always arouses considerable guilt among members of the suicide's family and in his medical attendants.

Greater medical awareness of depression and suicide, the introduction of antidepressant drugs and of natural gas, may all have contributed to the falling suicide rate. The Samaritans, a voluntary organization available at any time to help people in despair, may also have had some influence. Paradoxically, as the suicide rate has fallen, the number of cases of attempted suicide or self-poisoning has risen alarmingly. In 1970, one in five of all emergencies and one in ten of all admissions to medical wards was due to self-poisoning. Unlike suicide, women outnumber men by at least 2 to 1 and the majority are aged between 15 and 40. Barbiturates, tranquillizers and aspirin are the drugs most frequently employed. The act of self-poisoning is often an impulsive one, not intended to be fatal, expressing a variety of feelings, anger and aggression, threats and appeals, and often represents a way of escaping from an unpleasant situation.

Since 1961, when the Suicide Act became law, attempted suicide has ceased to be a criminal offence. It is now looked upon as a medical and social problem. But the problem, involving between 50 000 and 60 000 cases a year, is a huge one, and the area of responsibility is ill defined. Only about 20 per cent of patients seen after self-poisoning can be considered psychiatrically ill in the strict sense, although many of them are 'disturbed personalities', with considerable social problems. Adolescent female self-poisoners are likely to be promiscuous and to have had an abortion. A number of self-poisoners repeat their actions in the future, and not a few in fact do kill themselves eventually. There is an inverse relationship between on the one hand depressive illness and suicide, and on the other, open aggressive behaviour. During both world wars there was a sharp drop in suicides. And in Belfast during 1969–70, the suicide rate fell by almost 50 per cent and there was a corresponding increase in homicide and crimes of violence.

HYPOCHONDRIASIS

Hypochondriasis is a condition in which a patient is preoccupied with bodily symptoms and functions. Hypochondriasis is probably always part of another syndrome, most commonly an anxiety or depressive state, and is not a single aetiological entity. The incidence rises steadily with age and occurs equally in men and women. The commonest sites of hypochondriacal concern are the head, neck and abdomen and the commonest symptoms of these patients are pain, anxiety and depression. In about half the cases there is no obvious precipitating factor to be found, nor is there any physical abnormality to form a basis for the hypochondriasis. Nor are the patients characterized by any abnormality of their premorbid personalities.

However there is probably no one cause for hypochondriasis. Social factors frequently play an important role, and advertising is often aimed at arousing hypochondriacal concern. Sometimes hypochondriasis may be caused by doctors and nurses, although it is not so much what the doctor does which is harmful as the faulty way in which he explains the result of tests and investigations to the patient and his family.

It is important to recognize that although no cause for the patient's symptoms may be found, they nonetheless involve real suffering. Simple explanations that symptoms are due to increased muscle tension may be helpful but treatment usually needs to be directed against the underlying depressive or anxiety state.

14

SCHIZOPHRENIC ILLNESSES

SCHIZOPHRENIA

DEFINITION. Schizophrenia probably embraces a group of diseases, all characterized by disorders of thought, feelings and volition and a tendency to retreat from reality.

HISTORICAL. Throughout the 19th century there were numerous descriptions of what we now recognize as schizophrenic states, including what was known as 'masturbatory insanity' (believed to be caused by excessive masturbation). But it was Kraepelin in 1896 who first brought them all together under the term *dementia praecox*. He described the various symptoms in detail, but emphasized what he thought to be the crucial criteria, the progressive deterioration of personality which ended ultimately in a state of dementia.*

This gloomy prognosis was challenged by Bleuler in 1911. He introduced the term *schizophrenia* as descriptive of the splitting or fragmentation of psychic functions which occurs. (This must be distinguished from a 'split personality' which is described under hysteria.) He considered the basic fault in schizophrenia to be a disorder of the associative processes. He thought of schizophrenia as a group of diseases which, although likely to scar the personality in some measure, could remit at any stage without severe deterioration.

Bleuler's concepts are responsible for some of the diagnostic disagreement that exists today, especially between America and European psychiatry. In America any unusual psychiatric state is liable to be labelled schizophrenia. Indeed the term *pseudoneurotic schizophrenia* covers a range of what in England would mostly be considered to be severe personality and neurotic disorders. Today attempts are being made to standardize the criteria by which psychiatrists diagnose schizophrenia.

INCIDENCE. Schizophrenia is a widespread disabling disease. Between eight and ten people out of every 1000 born to day are likely to develop schizophrenia at some time in their lives. Men and women of all ranges of

---

* True dementia does not occur in schizophrenia. Formal intelligence remains intact, although the behaviour of a deteriorated schizophrenic may resemble that of a dement.

intelligence are affected. More than half the patients in psychiatric hospitals today have schizophrenia. It occurs in all countries and cultures. Although cultural factors colour symptoms, the basic disorder is common in every patient.

AGE OF ONSET. Schizophrenia typically begins in late adolescence or early twenties. However, it can develop at any age. The later the age of onset, the the slower the splitting of psychic function and the more the personality is preserved.

DIAGNOSIS. Since many schizophrenics exhibit protean symptoms, it is vital from the diagnostic point of view to recognize which are primary and which secondary. Bleuler distinguished between fundamental symptoms, present in every patient, and accessory symptoms which might or might not be present. Today most psychiatrists rely upon Schneider's 'first-rank symptoms' to distinguish schizophrenia from other functional psychoses. Schneider listed these as:

1. Certain types of auditory hallucinations, particularly the patient hearing his own thoughts being repeated aloud, voices arguing and criticizing his actions.

2. Somatic passivity experiences, such as outside influences playing on his body.

3. Thought withdrawal and other interference with thought.

4. Diffusion of thought, so that other people are able to read and experience his thoughts.

5. Delusional perception and feeling.

6. Impulses and acts experienced by the patient as the work or influence of others.

If one or more of these symptoms is present the diagnosis is schizophrenia.

SYMPTOMS. The onset of the illness may be acute or insidious. Symptoms fall into six main headings.

1. *Disorders of thought and speech.* The normal association of ideas become disconnected and it may be difficult or even impossible to follow a patient's flow of talk. It is curiously woolly and never quite to the point. Thinking is over-inclusive; the normal framework of conceptual thought is lost and irrelevant ideas are brought in. Sometimes he stops in mid-sentence and, after a puzzled silence, begins a different topic. One patient described this *thought blocking* as, 'they suddenly start up the vacuum gap'. He believed his thoughts were being sucked from his mind by other people. Some patients complain that their thoughts are shared and experienced by everyone else (thought broadcasting). At other times thoughts race through the mind so quickly that the patient has no time to speak (*pressure of thought*), or irrelevant ideas constantly intrude into his thoughts and cause total incoherence. In chronic schizophrenia thinking becomes empty and rather facile, although the patient may attempt to cover this up by reading and talking about philosophy or psychology.

Rational thinking is gradually replaced by *fantasy thinking* (see p. 8.)

dominated by his emotions. *Condensation, displacement* and *symbolization* occur. *Condensation* is a mixing of ideas which have something in common, regardless of whether this is logical. *Displacement* refers to the use of an associated idea in place of the correct idea. *Symbolization* is the misuse of symbols, due to abstract being replaced by concrete thought. For instance, a schizophrenic said: 'I've an elephant in my head,' meaning that he had a long memory. *Neologisms*, newly constructed words, are formed; a *word salad* is when these are so numerous that speech cannot be understood. The speech of a chronic schizophrenic is often stilted and strange. Writing is similarly affected.

2. *Disorders of emotion.* During the early stages of schizophrenia depression is common. Sudden outbursts of panic, bewilderment or elation may occur, but these lessen as the illness progresses. Once the disease is established emotional feeling becomes blunted (*flattening of affect*), and the personality appears insensitive and even callous. Social isolation increases as the schizophrenic withdraws from his friends. The emotional coldness and withdrawal may be 'felt' at the first interview. lack of emotional rapport, described as 'like having a pane of glass between you and the patient', is a useful diagnostic sign.

Emotional incongruity, the showing of feelings that are inappropriate to the schizophrenic's thoughts or situation, occurs in many cases. A schizophrenic described with a smile how a poison was being injected into his body during sleep. Another laughed as he described his mother's death. Contradictory emotions, like love and hate, may be felt simultaneously and result in contradictory behaviour.

3. *Loss of will-power and drive.* Together with flattening of affect goes loss of will-power and ambition. Patients complain of this in the early stages of the illness. A young man previously active and energetic may take to lying in bed until midday, gazing into space instead of working. Nothing gets done in spite of urgent demands. His appearance is neglected. Dirt and squalor accumulate. He feels changed, that his thoughts and feelings are not his own any more (*ideas of passivity*), that his identity is being lost (depersonalized).

Sometimes this loss of will-power is carried to extremes, resulting in *automatic obedience*. The schizophrenic does whatever he is told or imitates every word (echolalia) and action (echopraxia) of his interrogator. At other times he shows *negativism*. He disobeys all requests or does the exact opposite of what he is asked to do.

Catatonic signs vary from stilted odd mannerisms and grimacings to the most extreme and bizarre posturings. A curious change takes place in muscle tone. Limbs can be moulded into unusual positions (*waxy flexibility*) which are sometimes maintained for hours on end. Many of the strange postures assumed have a symbolic meaning for the patient. Immobility may suddenly give way to wild destructive outbursts.

Schizophrenic *writing* may reflect this mental disorganization. Mannerisms, changes of style, word salads, repetitions of words or phrases, curious punctuations and symbols, make their writings as difficult as their conversation to understand.

4. *Delusions and hallucinations.* It is useful, for diagnostic purposes, to distinguish between *primary* and *secondary* delusions. A primary or *autochthonous delusion* is an idea or belief which appears suddenly from out of the blue for no obvious reason and is immediately accepted as true by the patient, despite its obvious absurdity. One of our patients believed that the Pope was in love with her and was sending her messages. Another one suddenly knew that he was in contact with certain beings on the planet Venus.

A secondary delusion is equally as absurd to everyone except the patient, but develops 'logically' from the patient's attempts to understand his symptoms. He believes that his next door neighbour is interfering with his thoughts or will-power by 'a vacuum gun', or by rays through the television set, or by poisoning his food.

Delusional mood refers to a patient feeling that something is going on which concerns him but is being kept from him. A bank clerk had felt thus for several days and was growing increasingly anxious. Suddenly, while having supper with his wife, he knew that she was trying to change him into a woman.

Ideas of reference are common. The patient becomes aware that something said or done refers to him. A ticket inspector said, 'Good morning. Lovely weather for H-bombs,' to a young man developing schizophrenia. He at once understood this to mean that the ticket inspector knew that he was a homosexual and was warning other people.

Hallucinations. Auditory hallucinations may consist of indistinct background voices and noises, or be clearly audible. Certain auditory hallucinations, in the setting of clear consciousness, are indicative of schizophrenia. These are hearing one's own thoughts spoken aloud, or voices criticizing and abusing the subject. Generally they are unpleasant and may distress the patient if emotional feeling is still preserved. They come from inside or outside the head and tend to increase when the patient is unoccupied. From his behaviour, it may be apparent that a patient is hallucinated. At times he may answer his voices aloud.

Visual hallucinations are much less common but do occur, particularly when paranoid symptoms are marked. Hallucinations of other sensations can also occur. A patient felt the experience of being raped, smelt semen, and heard a voice telling her that she would become pregnant.

5. *Disorder of perception.* Perception becomes distorted because it is dominated by one particular emotion or idea. External objects and events are still recognized, but their significance or meaning is grossly distorted. An empty milk bottle lying on the ground was recognized by a patient to mean that he should kill his mother. It becomes difficult for the schizophrenic to separate himself clearly from his environment and other people. Schizophrenics, in the early stages of their illness, sometimes

complain that they are changing their sex or that they are becoming someone else. Strange hypochondriacal beliefs sometimes occur.

6. *Physical symptoms.* Cyanosis of hands and feet, and a greasy spotty skin are common in young schizophrenics. Menstruation may become irregular or stop, as in any severe mental illness. Loss of weight is usual in acute schizophrenia.

Formal intelligence, consciousness, memory and sensation are unaffected (but see also Atypical Schizophrenia).

CLINICAL FORMS OF SCHIZOPHRENIA. Schizophrenia may appear in many forms. It is still usual to divide schizophrenia into four types: *simple, hebephrenic, catatonic* and *paranoid.* These are briefly described below, although in clinical practice we feel that these subdivisions have little value. It is much more constructive to think of the disease in terms of prognosis and probable response to treatment (see p. 146).

Simple schizophrenia. This develops insidiously in adolescence or the early twenties. Apathy and lack of emotional response and drive are the most marked features. Hallucinations are usually absent. Many are undiagnosed and drift from job to job, and finally into vagrancy.

Hebephrenia. The onset may be equally insidious. The patient often presents with depression, even attempted suicide. Later, emotional incongruity and shallowness become more marked. He may indulge in outbursts of fatuous giggling or smiling. Delusions and hallucinations are usually present. The prognosis is poor.

Catatonic schizophrenia. Motor abnormalities characterize this type, either of generalized inhibition or excitement, associated with hallucinations and delusions. After a period of depression and progressive withdrawal, the patient's behaviour becomes increasingly negativistic. He refuses food, becomes mute or shows echolalia. Bizarre mannerisms, posturing and grimacing occur; a curious pouting protrusion of the lips (schnauzkamps) used to be seen in the past more often than today. Stupor develops in extreme cases. The patient is unresponsive to what is happening to and around him, although subsequently after recovery it is apparent that he was fully aware of everything done or said. His body may be still and resist all attempts to alter its posture, or it may become curiously malleable (waxy flexibility). At any time catatonic excitement may supervene. This is one of the few psychiatric conditions when a patient can be extremely dangerous.

Paranoid schizophrenia (see p. 148). Paranoid schizophrenia starts later than the other forms, usually after the age of thirty. Delusions of persecution are the prominent symptoms and the personality is often well preserved for many years. Sexual delusions are particularly common in women. These patients tend to be of a more athletic (mesomorphic) build than the other forms of schizophrenia. Paranoid schizophrenia in attenuated forms, without much personality deterioration, occurring in late middle and old age, is sometimes called *paraphrenia.*

ATYPICAL FORMS AND OTHER TERMINOLOGY. Acute psychotic disturbances, where both depressive and schizophrenic symptoms occur and the outlook for full recovery is good, are sometimes referred to as *schizo-affective* disorders. They are not always easy to separate from manic depression. But the presence of any first-rank symptoms of schizophrenia should help in the distinction.

The term *schizophreniform psychosis* is sometimes used in place of *schizo-affective* to describe acute schizophrenia precipitated by severe stress, accompanied by considerable emotion, where the prognosis is excellent. The term *typical* or *nuclear schizophrenia* implies by contrast a poor prognosis. Schizophreniform psychoses are characterized by an acute onset, vivid dreamlike hallucinations, and catatonic excitement or stupor, in a setting of clouded consciousness. Similar states have been described under the name *oneiroid psychosis*.

Patients may present a neurotic picture clinically, with phobias and hypochondriasis. In the U.S.A. these patients are sometimes labelled *pseudo neurotic* or *ambulatory schizophrenic*.

AETIOLOGY. The causes of schizophrenia are still not known. There are two main theories. One maintains that the progressive splitting of the mind is probably a biochemical disorder interfering with central integrative mechanisms. The other holds that the cause is purely psychological, schizophrenia being the result of *regression* to an early infantile level. Although there is no conclusive evidence in support of either view, we believe that an organic cause will sooner or later be found.

Some contributory factors are known.

1. *Genetic.* A predisposition to develop schizophrenia under certain circumstances is inherited. The chance of the child of one schizophrenic parent developing schizophrenia is between 10–20 per cent. If both parents have schizophrenia the incidence increases to nearly 60 per cent.

Identical twins possess the same genes. The concensus of findings of a number of schizophrenic twin studies is that 61 per cent of monozygotic twins are concordant, that is both twins develop schizophrenia. Corresponding studies of dizygotic twins found that only 12 per cent were concordant, the same as for non-twin siblings.

2. *Personality.* Typically schizophrenia tends to occur in people of *schizoid personality*, shy, withdrawn and over-sensitive. Of course, only a small proportion of schizoid personalities develop schizophrenia. But the incidence of schizoid personalities is considerably raised in families who have a schizophrenic member.

3. *Body build.* When schizophrenia starts in youth the body build is often asthenic or ectomorphic. A pyknic or muscular build seems to act as a 'protection' against the illness. People of this build who develop schizophrenia usually do so later in life, and there is less personality disintegration.

4. *Child–parent relationship.* The mothers of schizophrenics have been accused of being cold and rejecting towards the child. This is believed to be an important causative factor by supporters of the psychological regression theory. The evidence for this is weak. R. Laing has put

forward the idea that schizophrenia is a form of defence, adopted by the 'scapegoat' of the family. Bateson suggested the concept of the 'double-bind' parental relationship. The child is confused by one set of reactions in a parent conflicting with another. Thus a mother may hold out her arms to her child and say, 'Come and give me a kiss', but at the same time her expression and tone of voice are such as to repel the child. When he hesitates she says, 'Don't you love me?'

5. *Social factors.* The incidence of schizophrenia is inversely proportional to social class, being nearly ten times more common in class 5 (the lowest) than in class 1.

Schizophrenics are found in greatest numbers in the centres of large towns. One theory holds that it is the impersonal conditions of crowded urban centres which cause schizophrenia. But it seems more likely that this feature is due to schizophrenics drifting there, partly because living is easier and cheaper, but also because they are able to avoid making close personal relationships.

However, there is little doubt that social isolation is an important causal factor in the development of schizophrenia. Studies of patients who develop schizophrenia late in life show that a high proportion are unmarried women. They tend to be schizoid personalities who consistently failed to make any real friendships. As their near-relatives die they become increasingly isolated. Paranoid delusions gradually develop out of this isolation. The incidence of schizophrenia is highest amongst those who are single or divorced. A much higher proportion of schizophrenics, compared to the non-schizophrenic population, are unmarried.

6. *Biochemical and endocrine abnormalities.* Many schizophrenics show clinical and biochemical evidence of endocrine imbalance and abnormalities of body fluid constituents. Some are remarkably insensitive to huge doses of thyroid or insulin. This reflects the schizophrenic's lack of physiological, as well as psychological, adaptability.

A small group of schizophrenics, with *periodic catatonia*, either retain or excrete nitrogen in excessive quantities as symptoms develop.

Schizophrenic body fluids are toxic to some animals. Much work has been done to try to isolate a self-produced toxin, particularly one which might be related to an abnormality of adrenaline metabolism.

7. *Hallucinogenic drugs.* These include lysergic acid diethylamide (L.S.D.) and marihuana. Small doses can cause schizophrenic-like symptoms. It was hoped that the mechanism of action of these drugs would lead to greater understanding of what caused schizophrenia. But the resemblance between these drug-induced states and schizophrenia is not very close.

Precipitating factors may be of almost any nature. Physical illness, childbirth, surgery, head injury, drugs of the amphetamine or steroid groups, and emotional conflicts may all act as precipitants. There is evidence that many schizophrenic illnesses are triggered off by a 'markedly threatening event' occurring only a few weeks before symptoms first appear. But in simple schizophrenia the illness usually develops insidiously, without any obvious cause.

PROGNOSIS.   Good prognostic signs are:

1. Symptoms have been present for a short time only, preferably under one year. After two years the outlook becomes bleak.

2. There is still plenty of emotional response. Flattened affect is a bad sign.

3. An acute onset, accompanied by disturbed behaviour, is a good sign. A slow insidious onset and course bodes ill.

4. The less schizoid the personality the better the outlook.

5. A pyknic body build.

6. Age of onset after twenty years.

7. The presence of strong precipitating factors.

DIFFERENTIAL DIAGNOSIS.   Schizophrenia must be distinguished from depression, obsessional states, organic states, drug intoxications, hysteria and epileptic twilight states. Catatonic excitement may at first be difficult to differentiate from mania.

TREATMENT.   Modern treatments have enormously improved the chances of recovery and shortened the period of illness. Treatment should be started without delay, preferably in hospital.

1. Phenothiazine drugs such as chlorpromazine are used initially. The average dose of chlorpromazine is 300 mg or more a day. Phenothiazine drugs have completely replaced deep insulin therapy used in the past. Extrapyramidal side effects may need to be countered by adding drugs like orphenadrine or benzhexol.

2. ECT is given routinely with phenothiazine in some centres. But more often it is given only in the presence of depression, of catatonic symptoms of stupor or excitement, or where progress is slow.

3. Other effective drugs which may be used in place of or combined with phenothiazines in resistant cases include haloperidol, tetrabenazine, oxypertine, pimozide.

4. Lost weight must be replaced, helped if necessary by *modified insulin therapy.*

5. Institutionalism must be guarded against. Occupational therapy and the atmosphere of a *therapeutic community* are important. But care must be taken not to involve the patient too much in an emotional sense in group therapy and other forms of interpersonal relationship, as this may act as 'a threatening event' and retard his progress.

6. Leucotomy may be considered for violent chronic schizophrenics who have failed to respond to other treatment. But it is important to realize that such treatment is for the benefit of others rather than the patient.

SUBSEQUENT MANAGEMENT.   Although a proportion of schizophrenics will always need to be in hospital, many can now return to the community. Phenothiazines must be continued for the majority of patients if relapse is to be prevented. In the past many patients relapsed because they failed to continue their medication. Today, long-acting injections of phenothiazines have significantly altered this picture. Fluphenazine decanoate

(Modecate), given at one to four weekly intervals stabilizes the schizophrenic patient, buffers the effect of stresses on him, and so allows him to work and live with other people and lead a much more outgoing and satisfying life. Trials show that over 60 per cent of chronic schizophrenics relapse within about 3 months if Modecate is stopped. In many cases treatment may have to continue indefinitely.

The benefit of this treatment emphasizes the need for adequate community services to deal with these patients. If a patient does not keep his out-patient appointment he must be visited at home by a social worker or domiciliary nurse. Hostels, rehabilitation courses, and suitable work must be provided. If the present policy of switching the chronic schizophrenic from the mental hospitals to the community is to succeed, then the community must provide for such patients. Otherwise both they and the community will suffer.

Social factors are also of major importance. The schizophrenic must not be allowed to drift into social isolation. He requires some stimulation from his environment to remain in contact with reality. But he cannot endure strong emotional pressures, whether of love or anger. The chances of a patient relapsing are increased if he returns to a home where he is exposed to too much over-protection and mothering, or rejection. Such factors must be adequately assessed and dealt with before the patient leaves hospital. If necessary, it is better that he goes to a hostel than to his own home. Work is of great importance in maintaining morale and lessening the risk of relapse. If necessary the patient should be registered as disabled, under the Disabled Person's Act.

PROBLEMS OCCURRING OUTSIDE HOSPITAL

Medico legal. Occasionally schizophrenics become involved in crime, sometimes of a particularly callous nature. But usually they lack the emotional drive necessary for planned crime.

Sudden unprovoked assaults may occur, sometimes in response to hallucinations. An innocent bystander may be struck a violent blow. Murder occurs very occasionally, and the rare case of matricide is nearly always a schizophrenic crime.

If a discharged schizophrenic begins to behave aggressively he should be admitted to hospital for observation without delay.

Marriage and eugenics. A patient with schizophrenic symptoms or with marked schizoid traits is unlikely to marry. But for those who recover, marriage raises problems. A relapse is always a possibility especially after childbirth. And the chances of any children being affected must be considered. These problems should be discussed fully with both partners.

Childhood schizophrenia. The same disintegration of mental functions and withdrawal from external reality occur in childhood as in adult schizophrenia. But the symptoms in childhood schizophrenia depend on the stage of intellectual and emotional development the child has reached.

There is always a change of personality and *every* aspect of development is affected. The child becomes emotionally cold and withdraws

PSYCHOLOGY AND PSYCHIATRY FOR NURSES

into herself. Speech is lost or becomes babyish or may never develop. Incontinence, unprovoked screaming outbursts, continuous anxiety and negative behaviour may make the management of these children difficult. Deterioration is sometimes extremely rapid.

Childhood schizophrenia is probably made up of a number of different conditions. Some of these may be organic. Often it is difficult to distinguish mental subnormality from childhood schizophrenia. Physical treatment with drugs or electro-shock is of little value, although phenothiazine drugs may be useful in controlling behaviour.

The prognosis is poor.

PARANOID STATES

Paranoid describes the feelings of someone that other people are hostile and unfriendly towards him. Many people experience occasional paranoid feelings, particularly when anxious and in strange or new surroundings. They attribute to others the anxiety and hostility they themselves feel. If they also adopt an unfriendly attitude they are, of course, liable to make other people really hostile to them.

In some people *paranoid personality traits* predominate. They are touchy, humourless and suspicious of everything and everyone. In their marriages they show unreasonable jealousies, and they have few friends. Social isolation increases their paranoid feelings.

These reactions are understandable in terms of everyday experience. But *paranoid reactions* may occur which are not understandable and which are then considered to be delusional and abnormal. Many of these instances are manifestations of schizophrenia, but the personality may be well preserved for years and other signs of schizophrenia be hard to find. The terms *paraphrenia* and *paranoia* are sometimes still used for this type of paranoid schizophrenic.

Paranoid delusions may occur during depressive illnesses. These can be understood on the basis of the patient's intense self-reproach. He feels he is being watched by the police and is about to be arrested for his past wickedness. Paranoid reactions are common in confusional and psychiatric organic states.

Often it is difficult to say when 'normality' ends and delusion begins, and the patient may need to be seen over a long time. Paranoid litigants, for instance, who believe themselves to have been wronged, may spend their lives bringing court actions, writing to newspapers, Members of Parliament and so on. There may have been a basis of truth initially, but this has become distorted and lost. Yet in other respects they are 'normal' people.

Pathological jealousy unaccompanied by signs of schizophrenia or psychotic depression, may stem from a minor act of unfaithfulness by a spouse. This then becomes the focal point for the partner's sense of sexual inadequacy and is elaborated into almost delusional intensity.

Sometimes a sane individual is 'infected' by the paranoid delusions of a close friend or relative and comes firmly to believe them. This is known as *folie á deux*. When separated, the 'sane' partner usually, but not always gives up the delusional idea.

Treatment of paranoid states depends on the underlying cause. Often the patient refuses to acknowledge that he is ill.

15

PSYCHIATRIC DISORDERS
OF PREGNANCY AND CHILDBIRTH

DISORDERS OF CHILDBEARING

PREGNANCY. Emotional changes that occur in pregnancy are discussed on p. 60. Some degree of depression is not uncommon during the first three months and sometimes raises the question of termination. Nearly all such cases of depression clear up fully before term. When depression continues throughout pregnancy the likelihood is that the woman harbours strong resentment towards her husband, that she feels rejected and unwanted, and wishes she were not pregnant. Discussion of these problems is usually more effective than antidepressant drugs. Phobic anxieties may arise from mid-pregnancy onwards. Fears that she will be harmed or killed in childbirth, or that her child will be deformed,reflect neurotic conflicts. Sensible, reassuring discussion with a nurse or doctor can usually dispel such anxieties. Occasionally depressive symptoms occur in the last month of pregnancy and then tend to persist into the puerperium. Pregnancy occasionally precipitates a schizophrenic illness, and termination may need to be considered in the early months.

Pregnancy sometimes occurs inadvertently, while a patient is still being treated with psychotropic drugs. Particularly if there is a risk that stopping her drugs will cause psychotic symptoms to return, it may be necessary to continue them throughout pregnancy. Possible teratogenic effects must always be considered, and ideally no drugs should be taken during pregnancy. However, none of the psychotropic drugs in common usage are thought to cause damage to the child. The first weeks are the most vulnerable period for the foetus, and many women taking drugs are not seen until they are six weeks or more pregnant. It is important that medical staff should not arouse anxieties in pregnant women by stopping all drugs and making alarmist remarks.

PUERPERIUM. About 60 per cent of women have short-lived emotional disturbances soon after delivery, burst into tears for no reason, and worry about their ability to look after the baby on their own. Most of these 'maternity blues' can be dealt with by a sympathetic and understanding midwife, and they clear up spontaneously.

Women of strongly obsessional personality, especially with their first child, may exhaust themselves in trying to be 'perfect' in managing the child, and a vicious circle is all too easily established if the child reacts to her tensions by crying and becoming more difficult to manage. Tranquillizing drugs, as well as sensible advice, may be required.

A small number of women develop a chronic sense of tension and fatigue, phobias and emotional lability, which persist for many years, and may result eventually in marital difficulties. Many of these patients respond dramatically to one of the M.A.O.I. group of antidepressants.

About 1 in 600 women develop psychotic symptoms, beginning mostly between the second or third week, but (by definition) any time during the year after delivery. Depression may be mild at first and only deepen after discharge from hospital. The woman begins to behave strangely, to comment that her child is starving, that his bones are protruding through the skin, that her husband is unfaithful, and so on. Clouding of consciousness may be marked, with hallucinations and excited behaviour. There may be severe depression and the risk of suicide or infanticide. Schizophrenic features may predominate, but often there is a mixture of symptoms. More than half these women have a family history of psychiatric disorders or have themselves had an earlier breakdown. It seems probable that childbirth acts as a precipitating factor rather than causing a specific type of illness.

Puerperal psychosis may occur after any child, although the risk is slightly greater with the first. A breakdown after the first child may be followed by several uneventful deliveries. Or the first two or three children may be born uneventfully and the fourth precipitate a psychosis.

There is no relationship between age and puerperal psychosis. The probability of a second puerperal psychosis is about 1 in 20, but each woman needs to be assessed separately.

Treatment is similar to that of the non-puerperal psychoses. Whenever possible, mother and child should be nursed together. If there is a risk of infanticide it may be necessary to keep the child in a separate room from the mother until the risk is passed. It is often advisable to wean the child and stop lactation. Psychotherapy and support are important later in restoring the mother's confidence.

TERMINATION OF PREGNANCY.   The Abortion Act of 1968 allows pregnancy to be terminated by a gynaecologist, provided that two medical practitioners agree that (a) continuance of the pregnancy involves risk to the life of the pregnant woman or of injury to the physical or mental health of the woman or any of her existing children, greater than if the pregnancy were terminated; or (b) there is a risk of the child suffering from serious physical or mental abnormalities.

Before 1968 a psychiatric opinion was almost invariably sought, as pregnancy could only be terminated if the woman's life or physical or mental health were likely to be endangered by the pregnancy. Today psychiatrists see far fewer patients, and these are mainly referred by gynaecologists prepared to terminate but anxious to know the possible harmful effects of abortion on the patient. Of the women seen by psychi-atrists, abortion is recommended in around 70 per cent. Of those refused legal termination, only about 1 in 4 or fewer produce a live baby, and few of these keep the child.

Abortion produces little or no adverse mental effect in women of pre-viously stable personality, or who have good reasons for wanting it. On the other hand, neurotic and inadequate women may displace their chronic sense of depression and guilt on to the abortion and regret what was done. Women with histories of previous psychotic illness need to be carefully supervised, but the risk of relapse, provided termination is carried out in the early weeks of pregnancy and the woman is not made to feel guilty by the medical staff, is small. In 1971, 126 777 legal abortions were carried out, and the numbers are likely to continue to rise. Conflicts and anxieties among nurses who care for these patients are not uncommon, irrespective of religious scruples.

Sterilization may be recommended after termination, and carries few psychiatric risks.

16

PSYCHIATRIC STATES SECONDARY TO ORGANIC CONDITIONS

DEFINITION. Psychiatric symptoms occur when mental functions are upset by physical disease, toxic factors or physiological disturbances within the brain. They form two main groups:

1. *Acute confusional states (delirium)* are reversible, fully or partially, when the cause is removed. Diagnosis depends upon the presence of clouding of consciousness and perplexity. Frequently there are signs and symptoms of an accompanying physical illness.

2. *Chronic irreversible states (dementia)*. Initially there may be confusion, but frequently there is simply a slowly progressive dementia.

Although organic conditions are responsible for the psychiatric symptoms, these are coloured by individual constitutional factors.

ACUTE CONFUSIONAL STATE (toxic psychosis). Delirium may occur during the course of a fever, as a result of drug intoxication, or during metabolic upsets. This state is characterized by *disturbance of consciousness*. The patient is disorientated for time and place. His attention can be held, if at all, for a moment only. He is perplexed and unable to understand what is happening to him, or to separate real from imaginary experiences. All aspects of memory are upset. He is restless, his mood fluctuates rapidly from depression to elation, and terrifying dreams interrupt his sleep. Illusions occur. Fluff on the bed changes into little animals. Cracks on the wall assume the shape of moving faces. Nurses become enemies to be attacked or avoided. Frightening visual hallucinations cause him to panic and react violently. These symptoms are liable to be at their worst at night, for external stimulation, which helps to combat confusion, is then minimal.

In *subacute delirium* consciousness is less disturbed. The patient realizes at times that his perceptions are abnormal and tries to understand what is happening to him. But his thoughts and speech are confused and it is usually difficult to follow him. His level of consciousness and accessibility fluctuate a good deal and helps to distinguish delirium from acute mania and catatonia.

Confusional states last from a few hours to days and weeks.

AETIOLOGY. The common causes are:

1. *Infections*. Old people and heavy drinkers are particularly liable to

become confused. An illness which causes an alcoholic to stop drinking often precipitates *delirium tremens* (see p. 104).

2. *Metabolic and nutritional disorders*

(a) Endocrine disturbances, such as hypoglycaemia.

(b) Avitaminosis, particularly of the B complex. Wernicke's encephalopathy and Korsakov's syndrome are related to deficiencies of vitamin B1. Deficiency of vitamin B3 causes pellagra: dementia, diarrhoea, and dermatitis. Deficiency of vitamin B12 and folic acid can produce psychiatric symptoms with or without a confusional state. Folic acid deficiency has been reported during the treatment of epileptics with phenytoin (Epanutin).

(c) Cerebral anoxia, such as occurs in chronic pulmonary disease or heart failure; Confusional states resulting from impairment of cerebral circulation in heart failure rapidly disappear once circulation improves.

(d) Dehydration and electrolytic disturbances.

3. *Intoxication*

(a) *Exogenous factors.* Excessive amounts of alcohol and other drugs. Quite often old people, who may have become confused as a result of of infection or heart failure, are made worse by treatment. This is particularly so when they are given tranquillizers and sedatives or antidepressants. Other drugs which may cause confusion or psychotic reactions are opiates and anti-Parkinsonian drugs.

(b) *Endogenous factors* such as uraemia and hepatic failure.

4. *Miscellaneous.* Not everyone suffering from brain damage or infection becomes confused. There may well be an individual predisposition to develop a confusional state. Cerebral tumour occasionally gives rise to confusion. Post epileptic confusional states are relatively uncommon. Post-operative confusional states occur, particularly in the old, and especially after operations on the eye or prostate gland. The post-traumatic confusional state which follows severe head injury may continue for weeks and even months, fluctuating from day to day.

DIFFERENTIAL DIAGNOSIS. Clouding of consciousness and perplexity must be present for the diagnosis of a confusional state. Acute schizophrenic and manic patients sometimes develop incoherence of thought, but careful observation shows that consciousness is not impaired. Clearly the cause which underlies every state of confusion must be recognized as quickly as possible.

TREATMENT. Treatment consists of treating or removing the basic cause. Symptomatic treatment is very much easier since the phenothiazine tranquillizers were introduced; post-operative confusional states, for instance, can be treated in their own surgical wards. Chlorpromazine is probably the best drug to use, in dosages of between 25 to 100 mg three or four times a day. Care must be taken with old people, because of hypotensive side effects. If these are troublesome, thioridazine may be better. Haloperidol is another useful drug. In general, these 'major tranquillizers' are better than diazepine derivatives. They may need to be given by intravenous or intramuscular route at first. Barbiturates are best avoided, for all too often they increase confusion. After recovery, memory is usually hazy or absent for the period of confusion.

DEMENTIA. *Dementia* is a diffuse, irreversible deterioration of mental functions due to structural changes in the brain. The onset may be acute and initially disguised by confusion, or slow and insidious. As in confusional states, symptoms are coloured by the basic personality of the patient.

Although dementia is irreversible, some improvement is possible if the organic condition responsible for it can be removed; for instance, in general paralysis of the insane.

The incidence of dementia increases with age. If 'dementia' occurs in childhood it is then usually classed as mental subnormality.

SYMPTOMS. Loss of memory for recent events, particularly for names of people and places, is one of the first symptoms to appear. The loss extends steadily backwards into the past. A severely dementing patient may be unable even to recall his own identity. In the early stages *confabulation* may occur.

The dement can no longer see problems as a whole but narrows his attention onto one small part. Inevitably his judgement becomes faulty. His business fails or he is dismissed for incompetent work.

Initially, the dement tends to be irritable and emotionally unstable, weeping and laughing easily. Loss of emotional control sometimes leads to sexual difficulties. Delusions develop, usually of a hypochondriacal or paranoid nature. In the latter stages of dementia all emotional response is lost.

At first the dement tries to compensate for his failing powers by withdrawing from activities likely to prove too difficult. He develops a rigid pattern of behaviour, becoming excessively orderly and careful, repeatedly checking what he has done. He may suppress the knowledge of his deterioration from himself, or he may react to it by becoming anxious and depressed. When asked to perform a task beyond his ability he may react in a *catastrophic* way and break down completely.

Behaviour becomes increasingly difficult to control. He is easily provoked to rage. He becomes dirty in his habits, hoards rubbish, and wanders about the house late at night. He sets fire to things, turns on gas taps and forgets to light them, and needs to be constantly watched. Episodes of confusion, particularly at night or during a mild illness, are common in the later stages.

AETIOLOGY

1. *Senile dementia* (dementia starting after sixty-five). Senile dementia has an insidious onset. It may be noticed after an acute confusional episode. Depression in the early stages is common and responds to treatment. Death usually occurs three to five years after symptoms first appear.

2. *Arteriosclerotic dementia.* Arteriosclerotic dementia is not necessarily associated with hypertension, although signs of arteriosclerosis can often be detected peripherally. The onset is insidious, and the memory loss more patchy than in senile dementia. Emotional control declines but the

finer feelings of personality tend to be preserved at first. Depression and anxiety reflect the patient's awareness of these changes, and may lead to suicidal attempts. Later, as dementia increases, there are bouts of confusion and disturbed behaviour.

3. *Presenile dementias.* These are relatively rare forms of dementia developing before the age of 65. There are two main types, *Altzheimer's* and *Pick's* diseases.

(a) *Altzheimer's disease.* The usual age of onset is between forty and sixty years, but the condition can begin younger. Symptoms are the result of generalized atrophy of the brain.

Loss of memory is the first symptom. Fits occur in 25 per cent of patients, and the gait stiff, slow and unsteady, rather like that of a clockwork soldier.

(b) *Pick's disease.* In Pick's disease atrophy is most marked in the frontal and temporal areas of the brain. Mood becomes fatuous and jocular. Loss of emotional control may lead to anti-social behaviour.

4. *Huntington's chorea.* This condition is due to a single dominant gene, which manifests itself between the ages of 30 and 50 years. Symptoms result from atrophy of the frontal lobes and basal ganglia. Memory is often well preserved, even after several years. The first symptoms are rapid jerky involuntary movements, most apparent in the face and upper half of the body. Speech is also affected after a time and becomes difficult to understand. The patient is often aware of the significance of these symptoms and suicide is not uncommon.

5. *Secondary dementias*

(a) *Brain injury.* Dementia can follow on from the post-traumatic confusional state.

(b) *Inflammatory diseases:*

(i) All forms of meningitis, including tuberculosis.

(ii) Encephalitis. Dementia is rare, although personality changes are common.

(iii) Syphilis. Symptoms of General Paralysis of the Insane (G.P.I.) begin about ten years after the primary infection. Dementia is progressive unless the condition is treated with adequate amounts of penicillin. The different forms of G.P.I. described are mainly due to differences in the personality of patients. Considerable intellectual improvement can occur after satisfactory treatment.

(c) *Intracranial tumour.*

(d) *Avitaminosis,* causing beri-beri, pellagra, Korsakov's syndrome, Wernicke's encephalopathy, and pernicious anaemia.

(e) *Endocrine disorders,* such as untreated myxoedema.

(f) *Prolonged anoxia,* such as occurs in carbon monoxide poisoning.

(g) *Poisons,* such as lead, alcohol, and industrial chemicals.

TREATMENT. Much of the disturbed behaviour associated with dementia arises not so much from the organic brain changes as from the effect of the patient's surroundings on him. Indeed the majority of demented patients can and do remain in their own homes. Dementia in fact may only become apparent if the patient has to live on his own, is socially isolated and perhaps emotionally deprived. Although secondary dementia improves or is arrested by treatment of the primary cause, no treatment arrests progressive primary dementias. In old people in particular every attempt should be made to improve nutrition, large doses of vitamins be given if needed, cardiac output improved and so on. From time to time drugs are introduced which are claimed to improve cerebral circulation and metabolism, and therefore to help dementing patients, particularly those with cerebral arteriosclerosis. There is little convincing evidence that these drugs achieve much. Infection, physical debility and depression should be treated energetically but sensibly. The quality of nursing care of dementing patients is of the greatest importance. Much of course depends on whether the patient is treated at home, in hospital or in a special home. Occupational therapy is of great value and prevents or minimizes deterioration, particularly when combined with an active, organized ward programme of recreational activities. Dementing patients at home can be greatly helped by attending day centres, where there is an active social life and occupational-therapy facilities. Relatives need supporting, and a home help and visits by a district nurse are invaluable. It may also be helpful to take the patient into hospital for a week or two, from time to time, to relieve relatives or to allow them to go on holiday. Ultimately, however, it may be necessary to arrange admission to a geriatric unit or a geriatric hospital.

PSYCHOGERIATRICS

Psychogeriatrics is to do with the assessment, treatment and care of elderly people suffering from psychiatric disorders. About 10 per cent of people over the age of 65 (at present numbering $6\frac{1}{2}$ million) are believed to suffer from one or other form organic dementia, most commonly senile and arteriosclerotic. The incidence rises with age and is about 13 per cent in those aged 75 and over. The number of old people in this country is increasing, particularly aged 75 years and above. It is clear, therefore, that psychogeriatric facilities require to expand in the future.

Until fairly recently all forms of psychiatric disorders occurring in old age were included under the single term of *senile psychosis*. This resulted in functional disorders like depression and other functional states being confused with organic psychiatric states. Yet it is of vital importance to distinguish senile depression from senile dementia and confusional states. Senile dementia progresses and treatment is purely palliative. Senile depression, on the other hand, responds fully to antidepressant treatment.

Functional mental illness in the elderly, particularly depression, is still occasionally mistaken for dementia. Depressive illness is by far the most common psychiatric disorder of old people. It is frequently precipitated by a physical illness or disability. The clinical state is easily confused with dementia. The patient is slow, anxious, hypochondriacal, distractible, cannot concentrate and neglects himself. Symptoms respond well to antidepressive therapy. Care must be observed over the side effects of antidepressant drugs. Age is no contra-indication to ECT. If these patients need hospital admission they should be admitted to the ordinary psychiatric unit.

Schizophrenia of late onset (paraphrenia) is much less common. Women living alone are most likely to be affected. Isolation is an important factor and many patients have poor eyesight and are deaf. The personality remains well preserved. Delusions are usually related to unfulfilled wishes and are frequently of a sexual nature. One seventy-six year old woman was convinced that a policeman living next door was causing her to experience intense sexual feelings.

Senile dementia has been described above. The majority of patients are able to live at home; less than a fifth are admitted to hospital or go to an old people's home. The patient with mild dementia is liable to wander, is sometimes mildly confused and incontinent and may be noisy or aggressive. He does not need continuous nursing care. More severe dementia poses considerable management problems. But even here, a combination of day hospital and community services allows some patients to remain at home. 60 per cent of those requiring in-patient treatment are dead within 6 months.

Arteriosclerotic dementia. 70 per cent of those admitted to hospital are dead within 2 years.

Confusional states. Patients mostly either recover fully or die quickly. A small proportion go on to dementia.

A special although related problem concerns in-patients in mental hospitals who have grown old. Many of them entered hospital before effective methods of treatment existed and have become institutionalized. They have few or no relatives left, and it is more humane to let them stay in the surrounds familiar to them than to discharge them into the community.

PSYCHOGERIATRIC ASSESSMENT UNITS. It is vital to determine the relative importance of physical, social and psychological factors in any elderly patient with mental disorder.

Psychogeriatric assessment requires the co-operation of a team, a geriatric physician and a psychiatrist, together with the patient's general practitioner, social worker, domiciliary nurse and so on. Ideally a patient should be assessed at home or in the out-patient clinic, since admission to hospital itself is likely to provoke anxiety and confusion in the elderly. However there are patients who need to be assessed in hospital. Psychogeriatric assessment units are being established throughout the country for this purpose. Patients are fully investigated, intensively treated, and a plan agreed upon within three to four weeks for their long-term care and treatment if necessary. If further in-patient treatment is required, the patient is transferred to the appropriate psychiatric or medical ward.

TREATMENT. In-patient treatment requires skilled and sympathetic nursing, occupational therapy, and a well-organized ward routine and programme. Before discharging a patient it is essential to see that conditions at home are reasonable. Social isolation inevitably leads to progressive deterioration of mood and behaviour. Day centres are of considerable value for patients living at home.

EPILEPSY

DEFINITION. Epilepsy is a paroxysmal and transitory disturbance of brain function, causing characteristic electrical discharges, which result in a disturbance of movement, feeling or consciousness.

INCIDENCE. Between four and six people in every 1000 have epileptic fits at some time in their lives. The greatest incidence occurs during the first five years of childhood.

SYMPTOMS. Epilepsy can be divided into three types, all or any of which may occur in one patient.

1. *Grand mal (G.M.)*. A full G.M. attack passes through a series of stages. Many patients feel irritable and depressed for some time before the fit occurs. The fit itself may be preceded by an *aura*, which consists of flashing lights and other visual disturbances, forced movements, or peculiar sensations and emotions.

The fit begins with a generalized tonic contraction of all voluntary muscles. Air is expelled from the lungs, resulting in a weird cry. Consciousness is lost. The tonic contraction lasts up to a minute and is followed by a clonic phase of alternating muscle relaxation and contraction. This phase may last several minutes and during it the patient may bite his tongue and be incontinent. Subsequently the patient remains in an abnormal state of consciousness for some time. Repeated G.M. attacks in rapid succession are known as *status epilepticus*. The electroencephalogram (E.E.G) shows high-voltage fast waves or spikes.

2. *Petit mal*. Petit mal is less common. The attack consists of a sudden short interruption of consciousness. The patient breaks off a conversation or stops what he is doing for a second or so, then resumes where he left off. Sometimes muscle tone is suddenly lost (*akinetic seizure*) and the patient falls. Continuous petit mal attacks are known as *pyknolepsy*.

The E.E.G. shows spikes and waves occuring at the rate of three a second.

3. *Focal epilepsy* includes all epileptic phenomena, sensory or motor, in which the abnormal discharge remains localized to one part of the brain. From a psychiatric point of view the most interesting of these is *psycho-motor* or *temporal lobe* epilepsy; seizure manifestations include automatic behaviour, visceral sensations, illusions and hallucinations, dreamy states, and memory disturbances. Symptoms manifest themselves in a variety of ways. The patient may become confused, paranoid or aggressive. Unpleasant emotions, particularly fear, make themselves felt. *Déjà vu* phenomena,

159

hallucinations, unreality and depersonalization feelings sometimes occur. During an attack the patient may behave as an automaton, subsequently remembering nothing. Abnormal symptoms of smell or taste are fairly common, as are auditory and visual hallucinations.

PSYCHIATRIC ASPECTS

1. *Symptoms caused by epileptic activity interfering with mental functions.*
(a) *Directly related to the fits:*

(i) Depression and irritability may precede a fit by one or more days.

(ii) When consciousness is not totally lost, automatic behaviour, perhaps at variance with the personality of the patient, may occur. This *twilight* state can occur before, during or after a fit. Amnesia for the period of automatic behaviour is usually complete.

(iii) Delusions and hallucinations occur during *temporal lobe epilepsy* and may last several days.

(b) *Indirectly related to the fits:*

(i) *Paranoid psychoses* sometimes develop in middle-aged patients with *temporal lobe epilepsy.*

(ii) *Epileptic personality* formation. The epileptic becomes egocentric, hypochondriacal, moody, touchy, and liable to outbursts of temper. This may be related to long use of anticonvulsant drugs, or more likely to the psychological disadvantages of epilepsy.

2. *Psychological effects of being epileptic:*

(a) Epilepsy is still a social stigma, as well as a disability. Epileptics may not drive and cannot take a job in which a fit is likely to have dangerous consequences. Although an epileptic can register himself as a disabled person many employers are reluctant to employ epileptics. In the public mind epilepsy is still mistakenly connected with crime, degeneration and low intelligence. It is therefore hardly surprising that anxiety, depression and other psychological reactions often occur in epileptics.

(b) Some children with *petit mal* learn to provoke attacks by staring at a light and flickiering their fingers before their eyes. Others bring on a fit by overbreathing. Some of this behaviour is *obsessional*, some *hysterical*.

AETIOLOGY

1. *Heredity.* It is important to understand that any of us can have a fit if our brains are sufficiently stimulated. Epileptics only differ in the fact that their brains have a low threshold for discharging. Hereditary factors are important in 'idiopathic' epilepsy.

2. *Brain damage* is found, during E.E.G. investigation, in 75 per cent or more epileptics. Anoxia and trauma are believed to be responsible for many of these.

3. *Precipitating factors.* In young children, convulsions occur during fevers. Other precipitating factors are over-breathing, fatigue, emotional distress, over-hydration and hypoglycaemia.

TREATMENT AND MANAGEMENT.   In the past, epileptics were sent to epileptic colonies. This is now considered to militate against their recovery, and the policy is to maintain epileptics in the community. However, about 2000 people still live in epileptic colonies and are unable, for one reason or another, to return to the community.

Treatment aims firstly to control seizures with the smallest dose of drugs possible, and without causing side effects. And secondly to help the patient deal with the social problems which may arise from epilepsy. A number of drugs are available. Those in common use for the control of *petit mal* seizures are ethosuximide (250–1500 mg a day), and troxidone (300–1200 mg a day). For *grand mal* and *focal epilepsy*, phenobarbitone (60–180 mg a day), primidone (250–1500 mg a day), phenytoin (100–300 mg a day), sulthiame (200–600 mg a day). Sulthiame (Ospolot) is mainly used in the treatment of temporal lobe epilepsy. Side effects, such as drowsiness, ataxia, headache, are common and require the dosage to be reduced. Psychotic reactions have also been reported. Carbamazepine (Tegretol) is also used in temporal lobe epilepsy as well as for trigeminal neuralgia. In practice, control is often best achieved by a combination of drugs.

Intravenous diazepam, 10–20 mg, is invaluable in controlling status epilepticus.

There are about 60 000 schoolchildren with epilepsy in England and Wales. Provided their intelligence is reasonable (about 10 per cent of epileptic children are subnormal), and fits are not too frequent, these children should attend ordinary schools. Even when fits are well controlled, the epileptic child is especially likely to have difficulties in learning and in making friends. Puberty and leaving school are periods of particular stress. Special residential schools exist for disturbed epileptic children.

Adults should understand what happens during a fit and the risks to be avoided in work and play. Severe epileptics may need to be assessed in a regional neurological centre, associated with a workshop and hostel accommodation. Marriage raises the question of epilepsy being transmitted to children, quite apart from the difficulties that an epileptic may encounter in marriage. No general rules can be laid down and the matter needs to be discussed fully with both partners.

Psychotherapy of a general sort is helpful in dealing with the anxieties and behaviour disorders that may occur in epileptic patients. Parents, as well as their epileptic child, respond to explanation and encouragement. Temporal lobectomy may occasionally need to be considered.

17

PSYCHIATRIC DISORDERS OF CHILDREN

The child may be father to the man, but from a psychiatric point of view it is wrong to regard the child as a mini-adult. His developing, changing needs, personality and intelligence, his long and total dependence on his parents and other adults, both materially and emotionally, cause child psychiatry to differ in many ways from adult. Children react very quickly and often dramatically to emotional stresses. Their disturbed behaviour stops equally rapidly when the causes are removed.

Anxious parents may bring their child to a doctor for what sometimes seem trivial reasons. It is important that the person consulted is able to recognize whether or not a child's behaviour is within normal limits. It is also important for him to recognize that the parents may really be seeking advice about their own problems rather than about their child.

The child may be referred to a psychiatric clinic attached to a hospital, or to a child guidance clinic run by the local authority. Child psychiatric clinics are run by psychiatrists, while child guidance clinics may be staffed largely by non-medical people, under an educational psychologist and a visiting psychiatrist. Diagnosis and therapy are a matter for teamwork and close co-operation between child psychiatrist, psychologist and social worker. The psychiatrist, because he often has a broader view of the child, should head the team. The educational or clinical psychologist tests the child's intelligence by a means of special tests, and sometimes treats children, particularly when therapy is essentially educational—for instance, reading disabilities. The social worker is mainly concerned with the child's family and environment. Apart from gathering information which aids in the diagnosis, she will provide valuable support to parents during their child's treatment. Psychotherapy with a parent is sometimes undertaken by the social worker, under the label of social casework.

DISORDERS OF FEEDING

Disorders of feeding are a common expression of discord between a child and his mother. There is still a mystique associated with infant feeding. Although breast-feeding is no longer eulogized, some mothers still feel ashamed of not wishing or being able to breast-feed. Sometimes their shame is reinforced by the attitudes of midwives and practitioners. Such conflicts are likely to be most severe in women with ambivalent feelings towards their child, who have difficulty in accepting the role of mother. An anxious or resentful mother is likely to find that her child refuses to feed satisfactorily, vomits after feeding, and cries fretfully. Weaning, or a change to solid food, may be followed by negativistic behaviour. A similar pattern of events can develop if an infant is separated from his mother and fed by someone unfamiliar with his ways.

Infant feeding disorders, particularly among middle-class mothers, have probably lessened since the rigid routines once advocated became unfashionable. There is a wide variation in the feeding preferences and habits of infants and young children.

Abdominal colic, which can occur around the age of 3 weeks and lasts until the infant is about 3 months old, is frequently associated with an over-anxious mother. Such an infant screams nearly every afternoon for several hours. Screaming is only temporarily relieved by feeding. The over-anxious mother feeds her infant whenever he shows distress, thereby increasing the peristaltic activity of his gut. When the child is about 3 months old, abdominal colic stops as mysteriously as it started. It seems probable that the infant has some underlying physical predisposition, and that his mother's behaviour reinforces or activates this.

Regurgitation of food may be associated with slowness of eating. This can be an indication of resistance by the child to feeding, or simply a reflection of the child's temperament. But whatever the cause, regurgitation or slowness of eating causes anxiety and resentment in a vulnerable mother. *Vomiting* in the absence of organic cause is a more extreme expression of a child's disturbance. Sometimes it will begin in the setting of a physical illness, but subsequently pursues its own course. Maternal anxiety and resentment build up and result in the creation of a vicious circle.

Slowness of feeding, refusal to eat, or extreme faddiness may develop in a child for the first time at about the age of 3. Such behaviour is again often reinforced by the angry attacking reactions of his mother.

In contrast, over-eating in infancy and early childhood can arise as a reaction to a mother's anxious or rejecting behaviour to her child. *Obesity* in childhood is related to many factors, which include genetic and family attitudes towards food. In some cases a fat child's mother is grossly over-protective. She may be over-compensating for an unhappy marriage, or she may be afraid that he will die young as an older child did. An obese child tends to be physically lethargic, to be rejected by peers, to become increasingly dependent upon his mother. A vicious circle arises. The fat child of 10 or 11 is all too likely to develop into an obese adult.

Pica, the eating of non-nutritive materials like dirt, paint, plaster, is not uncommon up to the age of 3 or so, particularly when training is poor. But at older ages such behaviour is more often a sign of subnormality, or organic or psychotic illness, or of severe emotional disturbance. Lead poisoning is a possible complication.

EXCRETORY DISORDERS

1. *Nocturnal enuresis.* Nocturnal enuresis is one of the commonest symptoms encountered in child psychiatry. Although the majority of children are dry at night by the age of 5, up to a quarter of all primary school children are still wet occasionally. Training plays an important part in the child acquiring bladder control. Girls are dry sooner than boys. Nocturnal enuresis tends to be more common in some families than others, perhaps due to differing rates of maturation.

From the point of view of treatment it is important to distinguish primary nocturnal enuresis, the child never having been dry, from secondary nocturnal enuresis, developing after a period of dryness.

There are many causes. Organic causes include spina bifida, abnormalities of the urinary tract, epilepsy, diabetes. Organic abnormalities are more likely to be present if a child is also wet by day.

Familial and maturational factors have already been mentioned. Children who become dry at night at a comparatively late age may continue to experience frequency and urgency of micturition during the day for some time afterwards. Faulty training is sometimes responsible; a child may never have been toilet trained, or not be amenable to training if severely subnormal. Emotional problems are particularly likely to be present in children with secondary nocturnal enuresis. Secondary nocturnal enuresis may follow the birth of a sibling, a physical illness, maternal separation, starting school. There may be other signs of regression present, such as thumb sucking, disorders of speech or eating, insomnia. All these are usually short-lived unless deeper emotional conflicts have started in the child. Occasionally a very anxious child wets his bed at night when he is still awake. Frequency or incontinence of urine are then usually present also by day.

Psychological problems often develop in older children as a result of nocturnal enuresis. The child is afraid to stay away from home, and feels dirty and shameful. His relationship with his peers is then likely to suffer.

A child with nocturnal enuresis may wet once or many times during the night. Sleep is frequently deep and the child does not waken when he micturates. In the majority of children nocturnal enuresis disappears spontaneously. Parents should be reassured and a sympathetic tolerant attitude advised. Punishment is likely only to do harm, but a system of rewards for dryness sometimes helps. Restriction of fluids is generally pointless unless a child is drinking large amounts at bedtime.

Psychotherapy is mainly useful only in secondary enuresis. Conditioning, by means of a pad and bell, is successful in a fair proportion of primary enuretics. The aim of treatment is to produce awakening as soon as the bladders distends to the point of micturition. Micturition wets the pad which completes an electrical circuit, a bell rings and the patient awakens. In time a full bladder leads to the child waking before he micturates. If a child sleeps so deeply that the bell does not waken him 5–10 mg of dextro-amphetamine can be given at bedtime. The disadvantage of the pad-and-bell method is that it frequently wakens everyone else in the house. Co-operation by the child's parents is therefore not always satisfactory, particularly if false alarms occur. However, in cases of primary nocturnal enuresis, success rates of up to 80 per cent or more are claimed.

Probably the most simple and satisfactory treatment is the use of a tricyclic antidepressant drug, such as imipramine or amitriptyline at bedtime. For a child of around nine, 50–75 mg of amitriptyline is a suitable dosage. The drug usually needs to be given for at least 3 months particularly if neurotic problems are also present.

Hypnosis is still occasionally used successfully with older children.

2. *Constipation.* Bowel training is usually complete by the age of 2 to 3, with one or more motions a day. Not infrequently defaecation becomes the focus of conflict between a child and his mother, perhaps associated with other negativistic behaviour. If faecal retention is regarded as harmful by the mother she becomes increasingly anxious and resentful over her child's obstinacy; this in turn is likely to increase his resistance. Fear of the lavatory—a child of four may be terrified by his animistic thoughts about the lavatory—or fear of pain during defaecation due to an anal fissure, are occasionally responsible for constipation.

A child's attitude towards his faeces is conditioned mainly by his early bowel-training experiences. Children who have had coercive training tend to express hateful or fearful feelings. Children brought up more tolerantly enjoy the sight and feel of their faeces. Faecal play and smearing is normal in children of three or so. At later ages interest gradually switches to the faeces and defaecating habits of others.

Reassurance and discussion of the problem with the anxious mother and simple medical measures are usually sufficient.

3. *Encopresis* is the passing of formed faeces into clothing or other inappropriate places, after the age of three. There are two overlapping groups:

(a) Children with continuous encopresis since infancy who come from poor, specially deprived homes, and who have not been properly trained. Usually they are also enuretic and show antisocial behaviour. Many are of below average intelligence. Treatment involves habit training, perhaps in hospital, under a more consistent regime than is practised at home.

(b) Inhibited, obsessional children, mostly boys, who develop encopresis soon after starting school. They are generally deeply disturbed children, struggling with a rigid, tense mother. Soiling usually occurs as the child is returning home from school. Earlier bowel training conflicts between mother and child are reactivated, and constipation and retention overflow follow. Encopresis usually stops before puberty, but occasionally persists into adolescence or gives way to stealing and delinquency. Prolonged psychotherapy is necessary, and the child may need to be moved from his home to a special boarding school.

Persistent smearing of faeces over walls or floors after the age of three indicates anxieties and rebellion on the part of the child against parental pressures.

DISORDERS OF SLEEP

Sleep disorders arise when a child is anxious, or when family sleeping habits are erratic. But many two-year-olds resist going to sleep, or waken during the night, to make sure of their parents' presence. Angry parental reactions, or the parents' allowing the child into their bed, are only likely to prolong and intensify the sleep disturbance. Older children may refuse to go to sleep unless their mother is present, or may wake up and get out of bed to look for her. Elaborate rituals sometimes occur at bedtime. Such disturbances are rarely serious or prolonged.

Nightmares and *frightening dreams* can happen at any age, but are most common between eight and ten. The child wakens, remembers the dream and quickly loses his fear. *Night terrors* may beset children from any age from three upwards, but are most common between five and eight. The child sits up, terrified, in a 'twilight state' and cannot be woken or reassured. Eventually, after thirty minutes or so, he goes back to sleep. Next morning he is unable to recollect anything of the dream. Like nightmares, unless a frequent occurrence, they do not indicate serious problems.

Sleepwalking is common, particularly in highly strung children.

SPEECH DISORDERS

Disorders of speech can occur throughout childhood from emotional upsets. Speech may be delayed or, having developed normally, suddenly ceases or becomes baby-like, or stammering develops. Periods of stammering in childhood are quite common, about 1 per cent of the child population shows persistent stammering. Stammering is most likely to develop between three and four years, when the child's speech is rapidly developing, or around six to eight when the child starts school. Less often, the onset is at puberty. Boys are more commonly affected than girls, and several members of a family may stammer. Imitation probably plays some part in this. Parental over-concern and correction of the child exacerbates or prolongs the stammer. Severe stammerers are often inhibited people, but stammering itself is not necessarily a sign of psychiatric disturbance. Stammering can occur all the time, or only under certain circumstances when the child is particularly tense and expectant. Once the child recognizes his tendency to stammer he becomes more frightened of speaking (secondary blocking). Certain rituals and actions develop and are elaborated in an attempt to circumvent the disability. The chronic stammerer is inevitably frustrated, tense and insecure. He may react to teasing and mimicking at school by withdrawing into himself and his home.

Many stammerers spontaneously improve during puberty and early adulthood.

ANTI-SOCIAL BEHAVIOUR

DELINQUENCY.   Delinquency is a legal term. Children are only culpable from the age of ten onwards. Psychiatrists are often called upon to help the Juvenile Court, both as diagnosticians and advisers, and later as therapists. Acts of delinquency stem from many causes.

STEALING.   Stealing is more common in boys than girls by 10 to 1. Children who steal are more likely to come from broken homes and from lower socio-economic classes. Family attitudes and circumstances are strong contributory factors.

Stealing is often a group activity. The group generates excitement, and there is a need for its members to emulate one another, not to let themselves be considered cowardly. Stealing by young adolescents may be followed by mutual masturbation. Most children who take part in group stealing are psychiatrically normal. Often the group evolves into a larger unit, a gang, and at any time the group or gang may come under the influence of one or more disturbed children. It is then that serious anti-social acts can happen. Gangs tend to flourish in disorganized neighbourhoods, and in a sense represent an attempt by the children to create order out of chaos.

A child sometimes develops a compulsive drive to steal. The act of stealing symbolizes a need to 'prove himself', to gain independence and freedom from parental ties. Stealing of this kind is an individual act. Examination of such a child suggests that he is rebelling against a feared parent figure. Car stealing and joy-riding, by single, older children, tend to have a similar underlying motivation.

Another type of stealing, the 'comforting' type, begins at an early age, and stems from the child's feeling of separation from and rejection by his mother. Stealing gradually tends to spread outside the home, and to persist into adolescence. The stealing symbolizes a search for what the child feels he has lost. He is always insecure emotionally, only able to give or to take, not to receive. The act of stealing reasures him momentarily, and reduces his anxiety by putting him in 'control'.

NEUROTIC DISORDERS

ANXIETY STATES.   Children rarely experience generalized anxiety for long. Anxiety is usually phobic, attached to objects or situations which in themselves are harmless. The anxious child has difficulty in getting to sleep, is woken by nightmares, develops abdominal pains, headaches, sore throats, and may fail at his school work. He is over-dependent on his parents and becomes fearful when separated from them.

Single phobias are common in children; fear of the dark, strangers, going to sleep, animals, thunder, illness, a parent becoming ill and dying, vomiting, heights. The list is almost endless. These fears tend to change as a child grows. Fears and shyness reach their peak in middle childhood and then decline.

SCHOOL PHOBIA. The child with school phobia refuses to go to school. The peak age of onset in the U.K. is 11 to 13, a time when many children are changing school. In a young child, fear of going to school may develop acutely, but usually a child's anxiety over going to school develops gradually, particularly in young adolescents. Before leaving home the phobic child complains of feeling sick, headache or sore throat, abdominal or muscle pains. He sleeps badly and becomes increasingly withdrawn, tearful and dependent upon his mother. Eventually he refuses to go to school, saying that he is afraid of a teacher or of being bullied, of collapsing or becoming ill in class, of having to undress in front of other boys, of not wanting to eat school meals, and so on. In addition, the child often expresses fear that harm may befall his mother while he is at school. Once the child is allowed to stay at home his symptoms diminish. The onset of school phobia in adolescence may herald a severe generalized phobic state, but it is rare for psychosis to emerge later.

Boys (62 per cent) are more often affected than girls. In some cases there is parental discord at home, a mother compensating for an unhappy marriage by making her child excessively dependent upon her. But the older the age of onset of phobic symptoms the less likely this is. Treatment is often made more difficult because of parental collusion with the child. It is essential to get the child back to school at quickly as possible but this can take several months. Anxiolytic drugs may help to speed up his return. Often a change of school alone achieves success—sometimes to a boarding school. But a severely incapacitated young adolescent may ultimately have to be admitted to an adolescent unit.

About two-thirds of school phobic adolescents return to school after treatment. Follow-up studies show that while about a third of them become subsequently well adjusted, a third remain severely handicapped by neurotic difficulties. The rest show varying degrees of disability.

SCHOOL TRUANCY. Truancy is when a child stays away from school and conceals his absenteeism. This must be distinguished from school phobia, when the child stays away from school with his parents' knowledge.

Children who play truant are usually of below average ability at school. A high proportion have had learning difficulties and are retarded at reading and writing. They tend to be bored and unhappy at school. Truancy is frequently associated with other forms of delinquency. It has been repeatedly found that truants and delinquents share similar family and environmental backgrounds. Children who truant persistently can be brought to Court under the 1944 Education Act, and it may be necessary to send them away to boarding school if home conditions are unsatisfactory.

TICS.   Tics are impulsive, involuntary, repetitive, purposeless movements, like head-shaking, blinking, sniffing, shoulder shrugging, grunting. They occur most commonly between six and seven years, particularly in boys. Attempts to suppress the movements cause anxiety and increase the movements. If the child is left alone the tics almost invariably disappear.

THE AUTISTIC CHILD

Early childhood autism, starting in the first year of life, was first described by Kanner in 1943. When autism is present from birth the child is often unusually quiet and unresponsive to outside happenings. This may be so striking that the child is thought to be blind or deaf. Less often the child screams for long periods, for no obvious reason. Whereas the normal child of about four months lifts his arms and moulds himself to his mother when picked up, not so the autistic child. It is this lack of warmth and interest in other people which is so characteristic of autism. The child remains emotionally detached from his mother, and later shows no wish to play with other children; indeed he seems to perceive them as 'objects', not as fellow beings.

Speech development is retarded and half of autistic children never learn to speak. Of those who do speak, some use language for their own pleasure and not for communication. Many show echolalia and pronominal reversal: 'You' replaces 'I', and vice versa, and the child speaks about himself in the third person. Strange mannerisms, rocking, spinning or complex whole body movement occur. Obsessional and compulsive patterns of behaviour characterize the way these children play or arrange their possessions. They tend to become abnormally attached to nearby objects; if these are removed a reaction akin to 'separation anxiety' develops. Any attempt to change the child's routine or surroundings causes outbursts of rage and anxiety.

In general, autistic children are normal looking and do not appear outwardly to be unintelligent or subnormal. Boys outnumber girls by 4 to 1. Parents are likely to be of above average intelligence and well educated, with a low incidence of mental illness. But it is possible that this is more apparent than real, such parents being happier to accept a diagnosis of autism than of subnormality. There is no evidence of any relationship between childhood autism and adult schizophrenia. The incidence has been estimated at 2.1 per 10 000 with severe autism, and a further 2.5 per 10 000 with some features of autism.

Prognosis is best when speech develops by the age of five and when intelligence is at least average. Facilities for educating and treating autistic children are limited, and there is no certainty as to what method is best.

If the child is a disruptive influence at home, if other children are suffering, or if home conditions are unsatisfactory, residential placement is probably desirable. Otherwise it is usually better for the child to remain at home and attend a day unit.

The aetiology remains obscure. Psychogenic and biochemical causes, brain damage, or some inherent disorder resulting in perceptual learning difficulties, have all been suggested.

18

MENTAL SUBNORMALITY

The term *mental subnormality* was introduced in the Mental Health Act of 1959, replacing *mental defectiveness*. It implies a condition of limited intelligence, present from birth or early childhood, due to arrested or incomplete mental development. There are two sub-groups:

1. *Subnormality*, corresponding to the old term *feeble mindedness*, made up of individuals with I.Q.'s of between 50 and 70 (2.5–3 per cent of children),

2. *Severe subnormality*, made up of individuals previously labelled *idiots and imbeciles*, with I.Q.'s of below 50, who are incapable of leading independent lives or of guarding themselves against serious exploitation (about 0.35 per cent of children).

It is important to recognize that an individual is usually labelled subnormal, not because of a low I.Q., but because of additional physical disabilities, difficult or disturbed behaviour, or because he lacks a proper home. The incidence of psychiatric and behavioural disorders is closely related to I.Q. level. Children of 'superior' intelligence are more stable than those of 'normal' intelligence, who are in turn more stable than subnormal children.

Most children with I.Q.'s of between 55 and 70 are not labelled subnormal, and only come to notice in school because of educational limitations. They are then moved to schools for the educationally subnormal (E.S.N.); about 1 per cent of schoolchildren of school age attend E.S.N. schools.

On the other hand, if their behaviour is disturbed, until recently they were legally excluded from school and termed *subnormal*. Since April, 1971, under the Education (Handicapped Children) Act of 1970, the power to exclude such children from education ceased. Less than 0.1 per cent of schoolchildren come into this category.

After leaving school, the majority of E.S.N. individuals adjust well and become independent members of the community. Only a few subnormal individuals, with additional personality problems, require admission to hospitals for the subnormal. If unemployment becomes severe, however, the mildly subnormal are exposed and become a greater problem.

Most subnormal individuals belong to the 'normal' population, and make up what has sometimes been termed the subcultural defective group. Their parents are dull normal, or borderline defectives, mainly from social class V. Many are capable of marriage and of having children, although the number they are likely to have per family is less than the national average.

Severe subnormality is much less common. Among English children aged 10–14, the incidence is about 0.35 per cent, Mongolism accounting for about a quarter of the cases. Most cases of severe subnormality require, sooner or later, permanent admission to a hospital for the subnormal. Severely subnormal children come equally from all classes of society.

PATHOLOGICAL CAUSES OF SUBNORMALITY

Although it is possible to discover changes in the brain at postmortem of many severely subnormal individuals, in most cases the cause is either unknown or doubtful.

1. GENETIC CAUSES.   Harmful genes, dominant, recessive, or sex linked, are responsible for about 1 per cent of cases of severe subnormality.

(a) *Dominant genes* are relatively rare. A single gene is transmitted by a parent to (in theory) half his offspring. Fresh gene mutations probably play an important part in dominant conditions associated with severe subnormality such as *Epiloia* (tuberose sclerosis).

(b) *Recessive genes*. Both parents are carriers of the gene responsible for the recessive abnormality; they themselves are unaffected and fertile. Their offspring have a 1 in 4 chance of being affected. Recessive genes are responsible for such conditions as phenylketonuria, Wilson's disease and amaurotic idiocy. In recent years there have been considerable advances in screening and detecting heterozygous carriers of such genes.

Phenylketonuria is the result of an inability to convert phenylalanine to tyrosine, due to the absence of the enzyme phenylalanine hydroxylase. Phenylketonuric acid appears in the urine shortly after birth (identified by the ferric chloride test). Untreated, mental subnormality is usually, although not always, severe. Provided a phenylalanine-free diet is started within the first few months, mental development, in terms of mental age, proceeds at a normal rate. The longer the delay in starting dietary treatment the more the brain is damaged. It is still uncertain how long treatment must continue.

2. CHROMOSOME ABNORMALITIES.   Cytogenetics is a rapidly advancing study. Autosomal abnormalities are nearly always accompanied by severe subnormality. Sex chromosome anomalies can also cause subnormality but to a less severe degree.

(a) *Autosomes. Mongolism* (Down's syndrome) is the best known condition associated with an autosomal defect. Mongolism exists in all races and is the commonest disease entity in subnormal populations. In hospitals for subnormals, Mongols make up about 10 per cent of the population. The frequency of Mongolism at birth in London and the Home Counties is about 1 in 666, but falls off with increasing age due to the high mortality. Mongolism is related to maternal age. The incidence is less than 0.1 per cent below 35 but rises to 2.75 per cent at 45 and over.

Mongols have small round heads, slanting eyes, epicanthic folds, and often a convergent squint. Hands are square, with a single transverse palmar crease line, and there are characteristic dermatoglyphic patterns on palm and fingers. The little finger is frequently short and curved inwards. The tongue may be large, with transverse fissuring. Heart malformations are particularly common, but other organs are also abnormal. There is an increased incidence of leukaemia in young Mongols. Epilepsy and spasticity are unusual. Mongol children tend to be friendly and cheerful. They enjoy jokes, particularly at other people's expense, and are often good mimics.

Over 90 per cent of Mongols have 47 instead of the usual 46 chromosomes, the extra one occurring at chromosome 21 (trisomy 21).

(b) *Sex chromosomes.* Abnormalities of the sex chromosomes affect mainly the genital tract and do not generally reduce intelligence to a marked degree.

Turner's syndrome (XO) consists of dwarfism, sexual infantilism, and webbing of the neck.

In *Klinefelter's syndrome* (XXY), the extra X interferes with testicular development and affected individuals are sterile. They often have a eunuchoid appearance, with poorly developed secondary sexual characteristics. Their intelligence is usually but not invariably below average.

3. ACQUIRED METABOLIC DISTURBANCES

(a) *Kernicterus* may result if there is a marked rise in unconjugated serum bilirubin in the foetal circulation. Usually this occurs in cases of Rhesus incompatibility or in severe prematurity. Choreo-athetosis, fits, deafness and subnormality are likely to develop.

(b) *Hypoglycaemia* which is only likely to happen in very premature infants.

(c) *Lead poisoning.* Most cases occur between 18 months and 3 years, particularly among children from poor homes, and results usually from sucking or chewing objects with lead-containing paints.

4. HYPOTHYROIDISM

(a) Congenital absence of thyroid, unless treatment is begun within six months of birth, is likely to cause severe subnormality. Even when treatment starts at once, intelligence may be below average due to intra-uterine brain damage.

(b) Acquired hypothyroidism can result from the injection of goitre producing drugs such as phenylbutazone and para-amino salicylic acid.

5. BIRTH TRAUMA

6. PREMATURITY. Severe subnormality may be associated with a *very low* birth weight. Otherwise the suggested association beetween low birth weight and mild subnormality is probably related to the common factor of low social class.

7. INFECTIONS. These fall into two classes:

(a) Of the mother: such as rubella, toxoplasmosis, syphilis.

(b) Of the child: such as meningitis, and encephalitis.

CLINICAL SIGNS OF SUBNORMALITY

Severe subnormality may be obvious, or at least suspected within a short time of birth. The infant's appearance is abnormal, or the usual reflex reactions absent. On the other hand, subnormality is often not diagnosed until much later, perhaps after the child has started school.

When subnormality is at all marked *all* developmental landmarks tend to be delayed. The retarded infant does not suck, does not smile until late, is late in holding up his head, in sitting, crawling, and walking, in talking and developing sphincter control. As the child grows, his backwardness becomes more apparent.

The subnormal child lacks the curiosity and spontaneity of a child of average or above intelligence. Because of this he is often quiet and passive at home, and easy to manage. His speech develops slowly, his vocabulary remains relatively small, and abstract or conceptual thinking is limited. In the majority of cases there is no impediment of the senses, memory seems to develop normally, and although he may be distractible, the child's attention can be held by what interests him.

The presence of deafness, poor vision, marked spasticity, or frequent epileptic fits, still further limit the child's intelligence. A high proportion of severely subnormal children suffer from one or more of these conditions.

DIAGNOSIS. Diagnosis depends on the clinical picture, the mother's account of her child and his development, intelligence tests at some stage, and full physical investigations including biochemical tests and chromosome studies. The history must include a search for possible factors from the child's conception until birth and later.

Sensory deficiencies, whole or partial, aphasia, states of minimal brain injury, autism and psychotic conditions must be excluded as primary causes of the child's difficulty. In older children specific learning or reading difficulties may be responsible for a child seeming to be backward.

MANAGEMENT AND TREATMENT

1. *Parental reactions.* Very often a subnormal child's mother, particularly if she has already brought up other children, will be the first to suspect that her child is abnormal. Frequently her worries and suspicions are initially ignored or ridiculed. Later, when the diagnosis is confirmed, she is not unnaturally resentful and distrustful of medical opinion. But in many cases the diagnosis of subnormality is made even before the child's parents suspect, by a doctor or health visitor.

Parents should be told as soon as the practitioner is certain that the child is mentally backward. When the diagnosis is plain at birth it is still not exceptional for the mother to learn about her child through some casual remark by a nurse, or even from another patient in the ward who has overheard nursing gossip.

Except in a clear-cut conditions such as Mongolism, and even here there is considerable individual variation, it is unwise to make early long-term predictions about what the child will or will not be able to do. Rather, the parents should be told that their child will be slow in development, and will lag behind children of his own age. Terms like 'subnormality' and 'mental defectiveness' should be avoided, at any rate in the early stages. Most parents accept the diagnosis, and arrangements can then be made to follow up the child regularly and to give support to the parents. Occasionally parents refuse to accept the diagnosis and argue aggressively against it. Not unnaturally, some degree of depression and guilt, particularly in the mother, occurs after learning that her child is abnormal. In some cases marital tensions, which may have been present beforehand, are exacerbated and brought into the open.

Parents may overprotect their child or continue to deny that there is anything wrong with him. Much less often they reject the child, and insist that he be kept in hospital or transferred to an institution. A sympathetic understanding attitude on the part of the medical staff usually helps to resolve these problems; aggressive reactions can only make matters worse.

All too often there is failure to provide support and advice for the parents of subnormal children. Problems which are particularly likely to arise at certain stages of development should be anticipated; schooling, sibling rivalries, sexual behaviour at adolescence, and so on. Marriage is impossible for the severely subnormal, but it is not uncommon among subnormal individuals.

Genetic counselling may be required later.

2. *Treatment of the child.* A more enlightened optimistic attitude towards subnormality has emerged in the past decade. It is now recognized that many severely subnormal patients can be taught to read and write, and do relatively complicated tasks, provided such tasks are broken down into simple components, and they are encouraged and treated kindly.

The subnormal child needs a prolonged period of dependency upon his mother or mother substitute. Institutionalization is unsatisfactory but may be necessary if a child is severely subnormal with multiple associated handicaps, doubly incontinent, or overactive and destructive. In general, children brought up in large institutions are more retarded in emotional development, speech and verbal intelligence, compared to those who live at home. However, severely subnormal children, as they grow older and more difficult to look after, and children with severe emotional disturbances who are causing the rest of the famiily to suffer, sooner or later require admission to hospital

Most children with an I.Q. of above 55 are educable and will attend schools run by their Education Authorities. Children with an I.Q. of 70 and above, under the Education Act of 1944, are usually educated in ordinary schools. Those with an I.Q. of between 55 and 70 mostly go to special schools for the educationally subnormal (E.S.N.). Before April, 1971, if a child had an I.Q. of less than 50, and was thought to be unsuitable for education at school, he attended a day training centre until 16. However, under the Education Act (Handicapped Children) 1970, the power to exclude such children from education has ceased. All children now come under the care of the Education Authorities.

It is of the greatest importance to deal with physical abnormalities as early as possible. Epilepsy should be controlled with anticonvulsants. A deaf aid, or spectacles, should be worn without delay. Hormonal deficiencies must be replaced, chronic infections treated, and suitable diets and vitamins given where necessary. Physiotherapy will help to relieve spasticity. If a child's behaviour is constantly destructive and upsetting a phenothiazine drug will help to control this.

Even the severely subnormal child, when such additional disabilities are removed, can often be taught to speak, to read and write, to do simple arithmetic. Occasionally older subnormal children and adolescents who have glaring physical deformities improve in mood and behaviour after suitable plastic surgery.

19

TREATMENT

Over the past thirty years tremendous advances have occurred in the treatment of psychiatric illnesses. These, combined with changed social attitudes, have greatly altered the outlook for psychiatric patients.

Insulin coma, convulsion therapy and leucotomy were introduced between 1930 and 1940. Electro-convulsive therapy is still the most effective treatment for serious depression, but treatment by insulin coma is now virtually never used, having been replaced by phenothiazine tranquillizers.

The last two decades have seen the rise of psychotropic drugs, drugs which influence mental states and behaviour. Tranquillizers and anti-depressant drugs have multiplied and further advances can be expected in the future.

Psychiatric illnesses are now treated at an early stage, and vicious circles and bad habits are prevented from forming. But effective though these treatments are, they have their limitations. Often they only relieve symptoms rather than bring about a permanent cure. In the case of depressive illness, which usually 'lifts' spontaneously after a time, treatment may need to be continued until this occurs. But in some cases of schizophrenia there is no spontaneous remission, and drugs may have to be taken for many years, in the same way as a diabetic has to take insulin.

Each patient must be assessed individually. The majority need some form of psychotherapy or support. Physical factors, such as weight loss and/or vitamin deficiencies must never be overlooked.

After treatment, many patients require help to find a suitable job. Adequate *community mental health services* are essential at this stage otherwise the relapse rate will be high.

The following methods of treatment and care are described below:

1. *Drug therapy*:
   (a) Major tranquillizers.
   (b) Minor tranquillizers and sedatives.
   (c) Stimulant and anti-depressant drugs.
   (d) Miscellaneous
2. *Electro-convulsive therapy* (E.C.T.).
3. *Behaviour therapy.*
4. *Abreaction and narcoanalysis.*

5. *Continuous narcosis.*
6. *Modified insulin therapy.*
7. *Non-physical treatments:*
    (a) Hypnosis.
    (b) Psychotherapy and analysis. Group therapies.
8. *Prefrontal leucotomy.*
9. *Community care.*

TRANQUILLIZERS

A tranquillizer, by definition, has a calming effect on disturbed behaviour, without causing the muddled drowsy state that follows the use of sedatives like paraldehyde and the barbiturates. The term was first applied to the action of chlorpromazine.

Major tranquillizers or neuroleptics are those drugs which are effective in the treatment of psychotic symptoms. They act predominantly on subcortical structures.

(a) MAJOR TRANQUILLIZERS (NEUROLEPTICS)

Phenothiazine derivatives. There are nearly twenty different compounds, but they fall into three distinct groups. In their molecular structure they all share the phenothiazine nucleus.

Chlorpromazine (*Largactil*). Chlorpromazine appeared in 1952 and was quickly found to be effective in treating *acute schizophrenia*. Chlorpromazine, or one of its derivatives, often combined with electroconvulsive therapy (E.C.T.), has replaced deep insulin therapy in the treatment of schizophrenia. Recovery is better and quicker. The schizophrenic process is brought to a halt and the chances of chronicity and personality deterioration are reduced.

Chlorpromazine is particularly effective in *disturbed schizophrenic states.* Doses of 100 mg or more four times a day quickly reduce excitement and enable contact to be established with the patient. *In acute cases, of recent onset,* symptoms may be completely and permanently dispelled. *In more chronic cases* delusions and hallucinations may remain, but are now divested of emotion and cease to worry the patient. Such patients *must continue to take a maintenance dose* of chlorpromazine, otherwise symptoms will flare up again. This dose varies between 150–300 mg a day. It is no more justifiable to stop the drug of these patients than it is to stop a diabetic's insulin.

Chlorpromazine is also useful in other conditions in which there is over-activity and agitation; *mania, organic and senile states, post-operative confusional* and *psychotic conditions* and some *subnormal* and *psychotic children.* Up to 1,500 mg a day of chlorpromazine may be needed in some cases.

Chlorpromazine has no antidepressant properties, although in agitated states of depression it may be usefully combined with an antidepressant drug and/or E.C.T. Neurotic states, apart from anorexia nervosa, are not usually helped, although 10 to 25 mg three times a day does help some chronic tension states. *Obsessional neurosis* may be made worse, and hysterical symptoms sometimes become exaggerated. Large doses of chlorpromazine are useful in dealing with *drug or alcohol withdrawal* symptoms. *Delirium tremens* can sometimes be cut short or abolished if chloropromazine can be given intramuscularly or intravenously up to 100 mg, but it is an irritant substance and causes pain.

Promazine (Sparine). Some clinicians fear that chlorpromazine may cause jaundice (see below) and therefore use promazine, which is not hepatotoxic, instead of chlorpromazine, in the treatment of alcoholism. It has only about a third of the potency of chlorpromazine, and is *not* an adequate substitute in schizophrenia. The dose varies from 75–1500 mg a day, depending on the patient's condition.

Thioridazine (Melleril). Thioridazine is probably less effective than chlorpromazine in psychotic illness, but otherwise has a similar range of action. In doses of around 300 mg a day it has slightly less side effects than chlorpromazine, but when 600 mg or more a day is given for long periods retinopathy has been reported.

Trifluoperazine (Stelazine). Whereas chlorpromazine has a sedating effect, trifluoperazine tends not only to sedate by reducing anxiety, but also to increase available energy. Sometimes this stimulating effect can be excessive. Because of this double action trifluoperazine is often better than chlorpromazine in treating withdrawn *apathetic schizophrenic patients*. Trifluoperazine is also more effective than chlorpromazine in treating *paranoid states*. But if there are signs of agitation it is better to give chlorpromazine. The dose of trifluoperazine in psychoses ranges from 10–30 mg a day in two to three divided doses. Unlike chlorpromazine, small doses of trifluoperazine, 1–2 mg three times a day, are often useful in treating neurotic anxiety states, particularly in the elderly.

Fluphenazine decanoate (Modecate), *Enanthate* (Moditen). Long-acting injections of Moditen or Modecate have to some extent revolutionized the long-term treatment of schizophrenia. Modecate has largely succeeded moditen, due to its longer period of activity and lesser side effects. These drugs are given intramuscularly every 1 to 4 weeks, depending on individual responses. The usual dosage is 25 mg (1 ml), but doses of up to 100 mg may be needed occasionally.

SIDE AND TOXIC EFFECTS OF PHENOTHIAZINE DERIVATIVES. Side-effects are related to dosage, toxic effects to individual idiosyncracies.

1. *Autonomic and endocrine effects*. Dizziness and fainting due to postural hypotension, dry mouth, blurred vision, lachrymation, facial pallor, constipation and pyrexia may occur. These effects sometimes disappear as treatment continues. Menstrual irregularities and lactation are occasionally seen. Thioridazine in particular is liable to cause impotence.

2. *Neurological effects* are more common with trifluoperazine and fluphenazine, members of the piperazine group of phenothiazines. Parkinsonism, with rigidity, tremor and salivation; akathisia or motor restlessness;

akinetic or drop attacks, and dyskinesia resulting in spasm of groups of muscles, commonly of the face and mouth, the limbs and the back. These symptoms usually disappear when the drug is stopped but may persist if large doses of the drug have been given for a long time, particularly to patients with pre-existent brain damage. Epileptic fits may be provoked, particularly when large doses are first given, or if the drug is suddenly stopped.

3. *Toxic or hypersensitivity effects*. Erythematous and urticarial skin rashes occur and there may be increased sensitivity to sunlight with chlorpromazine. Patients should always be warned of this risk.

Jaundice occasionally occurs with chlorpromazine. It is unrelated to dosage and usually disappears when the drug is stopped.

Agranulocytosis is a rare complication.

Depression, and even suicide, have been reported with all the phenothiazines, but particularly with long-acting fluphenazine. This is most likely in well-preserved schizophrenics and in patients with schizoaffective disorders. Confusional episodes may occasionally occur and very rarely phenothiazines can cause, paradoxically, a state of excitement.

Phenothiazine drugs can be safely given with other drugs or E.C.T., but it should be remembered that they will potentiate the effects of sedative drugs, including alcohol.

Overdosage causes drowsiness, extrapyramidal effects and convulsions, hypotension and hypothermia. A stomach washout should be given, the patient kept flat and noradrenaline administered if severe hypotension persists.

Oxypertine (Integrin). In doses of up to 120 mg a day oxypertine will stimulate some apathetic withdrawn schizophrenic patients. It is also used in the treatment of anxiety in doses of 10 mg two or three times a day. Side effects include extrapyramidal symptoms.

Reserpine (Serpasil), is now rarely used, mainly because of the danger of its precipitating depression. In addition it is dangerous to combine reserpine with E.C.T.

Butyrophenones such as *haloperidal* (Serenace). This is a most effective drug in controlling *manic* and *hypomanic states*. It is also useful in chronic schizophrenia which has responded poorly to treatment with phenothiazines particularly when this is accompanied by auditory hallucinations. In acute states 5–20 mg intravenously or intramuscularly can be given six-hourly until symptoms are controlled. The oral dose varies from 1.5–12 mg or more two or three times a day. Small doses, 0.5 mg three times a day, are useful in controlling anxiety, especially in older patients.

Side effects. Extrapyramidal effects are common, but respond to anti-Parkinsonian drugs. Blood pressure is not lowered to any significant degree.

Thioxanthine derivatives provide a parallel series of psychotropic drugs to the phenothiazines.

Flupenthixol is probably the most potent member of the series and is used in the treatment of schizophrenia. In a long acting form (Depixol), 40–80 mg is probably comparable to 25 mg Modecate. However, comparative trials are still in progress. Side effects are somewhat similar to the phenothiazines.

Diphenyl butylpiperidines. Pimozide (Orap) is a relatively new drug introduced for the treatment of schizophrenia, particularly when associated with apathy. One dose only a day between 2 and 10 mg, need be given and has few extrapyramidal and autonomic side effects. It is a dopamine antagonist in its biochemical activity.

(b) MINOR TRANQUILLIZERS

These drugs have useful anxiolytic properties and have largely replaced barbiturates in the treatment of anxiety states. They have no place in the primary treatment of psychotic illness, although they may be combined with antidepressants and major tranquillizers in order to reduce secondary anxiety. Their action is probably mediated through the limbic system.

The *benzodiazepine derivatives* are widely prescribed. These are six compounds: chlordiazepoxide (Librium), diazepam (Valium), oxazepam (Serenid), medazepan (Nobrium), nitrazepam (Mogadon), lorazepam

TABLE 19.1

Drug	Usual dosage range	Parenteral dosage
Chlordiazepoxide	5–30 mg t.d.s.	100–1000 mg
Diazepam	2–30 mg t.d.s.	10–50 mg
Oxazepam	10–30 mg t.d.s.	—
Medazepam	10–30 mg t.d.s.	—
Lorazepam	1–5 mg t.d.s.	—
Potassium chlorazepate	15–30 mg t.d.s.	—
Nitrazepam	5–15 mg o.n.	—

(Ativan). Chlordiazepoxide and oxazepam are less sedating than diazepam and medazepam, dose for dose. Chlordiazepoxide can be given intramuscularly. Doses of 100 mg or more a day are used in treating *delirium tremens* and *alcohol withdrawal*. Diazepam may also be given intravenously and is valuable in the treatment of *status epilepticus* and in certain phobic states. Nitrazepam is mainly used as a hypnotic.

Benzodiazepine derivatives are relatively safe drugs. Overdosage rarely results in death. Dependence is also uncommon but is still possible. The main side effects are tiredness and drowsiness. Less usual are ataxia, headache, unsteadiness, and rarely (mainly in old people) confusion and hallucinations. They potentiate other drugs, including alcohol, and people who drive should always be warned of this.

Meprobamate. Meprobamate preceded the benzodiazepines but has now been largely superseded by them. 200–400 mg three times a day reduces anxiety. The disadvantage of the drug is that it is liable to cause dependence, and that serious idiosyncratic reactions can develop within 48 hours. These include dermatitis, headache, gastro-intestinal disturbances, purpura and cardiovascular collapse. Chronic intoxication results in confusion and ataxia. Sudden stopping of the drug can cause epileptic fits.

Benzoctamine (Tacitin), had a structure resembling the benzodiazepines. 10 mg three times a day lessens anxiety. Side effects are similar to the benzodiazepines.

Hypnotics and sedatives. The most popular sedative at present is nitrazepam.

Barbiturates. They are effective in reducing anxiety, cheap and have few side effects. The disadvantage is the ease with which they may be used for suicide, or cause habituation and dependence.

(i) *Long-acting. Phenobarbitone.* The main use of phenobarbitone is in epilepsy, 60–180 mg a day. Phenobarbitone is ineffective as a hypnotic at night. It should never be given to depressed, agitated patients, as it is liable to increase depression.

(ii) *Medium-acting. Sodium amylobarbitone* (Sodium amytal). 200–400 mg is an effective hypnotic dose. 60 mg, two or three times a day, is an anxiolytic dosage.

(iii) *Short- and quick-acting. Quinalbarbitone sodium* (Seconal). 100 mg acts as a hypnotic. 50 mg of quinalbarbitone quickly reduces anxiety. It is therefore a particularly useful drug for phobic patients to carry with them in case of panic, or for someone who fears facing an anxiety-provoking situation. *Methohexitone sodium,* (Brietal), 50–100 mg, or *thiopentone* (Pentothal) 250–500 mg, slowly given intravenously, is sometimes used to produce an 'abreaction'.

Side effects. The regular use of large doses of barbiturates is liable to cause confusion, unsteadiness and slurred speech and may increase rather than reduce tension. Sudden stoppage can precipitate a series of epileptic fits.

Bromides were at one time popular sedatives. Hypnotics containing bromides, such as Carbromal, are still available. They are best avoided because of the serious consequences of bromide intoxication, which causes confusion and psychiatric symptoms.

Paraldehyde. 10 to 15 ml of paraldehyde given intramuscularly is still one of the quickest and most effective ways of calming a violent patient. It is still given occasionally as a hypnotic, 8 to 10 ml by mouth at night. Although effective, its unpleasant fishy taste and lingering smell greatly reduces its usefulness. Intramuscular injection is very painful and can result in abscess formation. Some psychiatrists use paraldehyde regularly for controlling delirium tremens.

Chloral hydrate has a rapid short-lived hypnotic effect and is a useful drug to take on going to bed. The usual dose is 1 to 2 g. It has an unpleasant burning taste and is best mixed with fruit juice or milk. Chloral is broken down in the liver and kidneys to the active metabolite trichlorethanol triclofos (Tricloryl). It is also broken down to trichlorethanol; this is available in tablets of 500 mg each. Dichloralphenazone (Welldorm) is a combination of chloral with phenazone. One or more tablets of 650 mg produce sleep.

Other non-barbiturate hypnotics include *glutethamide* (Doriden) and *methaqualone* (Mellsil); the last is sometimes combined with an antihistamine in the form of Mandrax. Mandrax is included in Schedule 2 of the Misuse of Drugs Act which came into force in July, 1973.

Chlormethiazole (Heminevrin). This drug is used in the treatment of delirium tremens and of alcohol and other drug-withdrawal states, sometimes combined with chlorpromazine. Doses of up to 10 g or more orally a day may be required. The drug can also be given by intravenous infusion. Chlormethiazole will also damp down anxiety, and 0.5–2 g. is a useful hypnotic, particularly in older patients who complain of initial insomnia, and who are liable to become confused or seriously hypotensive on other drugs. Side effects are few. The main ones are sneezing and rhinorrhoea, headache, and gastrointestinal upsets. Dependence can develop and care is needed in this respect.

(c) STIMULANTS

Amphetamine and its compounds (Dexedrine). There are a number of drugs which stimulate the nervous system and increase alertness and speed of reaction. Amphetamine was introduced in 1936 to combat depression. The drug increases alertness, self-confidence, energy, and feelings of well being. At the same time appetite and the need for sleep are reduced.

Amphetamine compounds are still used by healthy people to combat tiredness and to reduce appetite and weight. They are still prescribed for people with mild depressive states, although they are now included in Schedule 2 of the Misuse of Drugs Act. But the value of these drugs in seriously depressed patients is virtually nil. The cheerfulness is transitory and often followed by increased depression. Also tolerance develops rapidly, the dose has to be increased and after about a fortnight's use there is no longer much effect.

Side-effects include anxiety and restlessness. For this reason a short-acting barbiturate, 30 mg amylobarbitone is sometimes added to the stimulant (Drinamyl). This has a pronounced euphoric effect in some patients. Doses of amphetamine greater than 50 mg a day can cause psychotic-like symptoms.

Specific anti-depressant drugs. These drugs represent a great advance in the treatment of depression, particularly of the milder forms. They have not superseded ECT, although they may reduce the number of ECT's required and lessen the chances of relapse later. Antidepressant drugs must be continued until spontaneous remission of depression occurs. They suppress but do not cure the illness, which in most instances is a self-limiting disease. If the antidepressant is reduced or stopped too soon, symptoms quickly reappear. Therapeutic effects may take up to a fortnight or more to appear, and six to eight weeks to reach maximum effectiveness. Side effects on the other hand develop almost immediately. Drug dosage varies enormously from one patient to another. The effectiveness of the drug depends on its steady-state plasma level, and people differ widely in the rate at which they metabolize, absorb, and excrete these drugs. A patient who metabolizes say imipramine slowly may only require 30 mg a day, while another patient who rapidly metabolizes the drug may need up to 600 mg a day.

There are two separate groups of antidepressant drugs; the tricyclic antidepressants and the monoamine oxidase inhibitors (M.A.O.I.).

TABLE 19.2

Drug	Daily dosage range	Sedating properties	Anticholinergic effects
Imipramine	30–600 mg	—	+++
Clomipramine	30–600 mg	—	+++
Amitriptyline	30–600 mg	++	++
Nortriptyline	30–200 mg	++	+
Desipramine	30–600 mg	+	++
Trimipramine	30–600 mg	+++	+
Protriptyline	10–80 mg	—	+
Iprindole	45–135 mg	—	—
Dothiepin	50–300 mg	+	+
Doxepin	30–600 mg	++	+
Dibenzepin	80–480 mg	+	+

Both were introduced at about the same time, in the later 1950s. The tricyclics have a greater range of activity than the M.A.O.I.'s and are less likely to cause toxic effects.

The *tricyclic antidepressants* are most effective in the more endogenous type of depression, with early morning waking, loss of appetite and weight and so on. It is important to remember that depression of mood may be absent, and that 'masked depressions' are common. Imipramine was the first of many analogues to be introduced. All these drugs act by preventing the uptake of monoamines at the synaptic cleft, and thus increasing the concentration of these substances in certain areas of the brain (see p. 72), some are more sedating, others more stimulating.

It is often best to give all or most of the more sedating antidepressant compounds at bedtime. Not only does the patient then feel less sleepy in the daytime, but insomnia is countered. Combinations of other drugs with the antidepressants may be necessary. Tranquillizers like the pheno-thiazines inhibit the metabolism of tricyclic drugs by influencing the liver enzymes, and therefore are liable to increase antidepressant plasma levels. Barbiturates, on the other hand, increase the rate of breakdown of a tricyclic antidepressant and therefore lower its plasma level. Alcohol has a similar lowering effect.

Side effects can be troublesome, particularly in old people. Those arising from the anticholinergic properties of the drug are dry mouth, tachycardia, hypotension, constipation, difficulty in micturition, blurring of vision and a liability to aggravate glaucoma, impotence or an inability to achieve orgasm. Sweating over the upper half of the body can be profuse. Muscular side effects include a fine tremor, increased reflexes, and occasionally drop attacks. Epileptic tendencies may be increased. Confusion and hallucinations, usually visual, occur mainly in older patients, and especially at night. Electrocardiographic changes may occur. S.T. segments are depressed, T-waves flattened and Q.T. intervals prolonged. Amitriptyline has been reported to cause cardiac irregularities and death in patients with already diseased hearts. There is no evidence that any of these drugs have teratogenic effects in humans.

Monoamine oxidase inhibitors (M.A.O.I.). The M.A.O.I.'s have a narrower range of usefulness, but are invaluable in treating reactive or neurotic forms of depression, especially when these are accompanied by phobic anxiety. Many of the patients who become 'neurotic invalids' after childbirth, having previously coped well with their responsibilities, respond dramatically to an M.A.O.I., often combined with a tranquillizer. All these drugs act by inhibiting monoamine oxidase, which normally destroys monoamines released into the synaptic clefts. The concentration of these substances therefore increases at these sites.

Iproniazid (Marsilid) was the first M.A.O.I. to be used in psychiatry (1957). It was very effective, but because liver damage sometimes followed its use less toxic analogues were produced. These include *phenelzine* (Nardil), *isocarboxazide* (Marplan), *nialamide* (Niamid), *methylbenzyl-hydrazine* (Actomol) and *tranylcypromine* (Parnate).

Dosage. The equivalent dosage of the M.A.O.I. drugs is shown below:

Nardil	1 tablet (15 mg),	3-4 times a day.
Marplan	1 tablet (10 mg),	3-4 times a day.
Niamid	2 tablets (50 mg),	3-4 times a day.
Parnate	1 tablet (10 mg),	2-4 times a day.

Side-effects are numerous and include dizziness due to postural hypotension, dry mouth, constipation, difficulty in starting micturition, loss of sexual potency, ankle oedema, muscle twitchings and jerking at night, peripheral neuritis, anaemia, and a reduced need for sleep. Manic, schizophrenic and confusional states may occur if patients are not well selected and supervised. Jaundice, sometimes fatal, has been reported after the use of all the M.A.O.I.'s except Parnate.

A severe pounding occipital headache, which may be mistaken for a subarachnoid haemorrhage, occurs with too high a dosage, or when an M.A.O.I. is combined with certain foodstuffs containing tyramine, such as cheese, yoghurt, Marmite, Bovril, and heavy beers. Normally tyramine is broken down in the wall of the gut. But when a patient is taking an M.A.O.I., tyramine is absorbed directly into the blood stream where it may release catechol amines. This results in what is known as a *hypertensive crisis*, with a rapid rise of blood pressure. Symptoms start half an hour or so after the meal, with palpitations and painful throbbing in the neck and occipital area which rapidly becomes excruciating and generalized. Reaction may last from half to several hours. Deaths have occasionally occurred. M.A.O.I.'s potentiate the effects of alcohol and other drugs, particularly morphine and pethidine. Hypertensive reactions occur if an M.A.O.I. is given to a patient receiving methyldopa (Aldomet), L-dopa, and some tricyclic compounds. Patients who fail to respond to treatment with individual antidepressants and/or E.C.T. sometimes do so when a M.A.O.I. and a tricyclic are combined. Trimipramine, amitriptyline, and nortriptyline, the more sedating compounds, can be combined with an M.A.O.I. with little risk of a hypertensive crisis. If a hypertensive crisis should occur, phenotolamine (5 mg) should be given intravenously as quickly as possible.

OTHER DRUGS USED IN DEPRESSIVE ILLNESS

Lithium salts. Lithium salts are highly effective in preventing manic depressive attacks. They are also useful in the treatment of acute mania, although not as good as chlorpromazine or haloperidol. Lithium carbonate (Camcolit) is now given regularly to patients with established attacks of manic depression. The drug is given orally and the dose is adjusted until the serum lithium concentration lies between 0.8 to 1.2 ml Eq per litre. Blood should be taken for testing 12 hours after the last dose, otherwise false readings are liable to be obtained. The drug must be continued for many years, perhaps for ever, if attacks are to be prevented or effectively reduced in frequency and intensity. The drug replaces intracellular sodium, but its exact mode of action is unknown. Early side effects include a fine tremor, nausea, vomiting, diarrhoea and tiredness, but these often disappear after a few weeks, or if the drug is given in slow release form (Priadel). Toxic effects occur if the serum lithium level reaches 2 mlEq/l or more. Severe nausea and diarrhoea, coarse tremor, ataxia and dizziness, polyuria and polydipsia are indications for immediately stopping the drug. Skin rashes are uncommon. Diffuse non-toxic goitres are quite common in patients who have been on lithium for a long time. There is no evidence of teratogenic effects in man.

Thyroxine is said to potentiate the effect of tricyclic antidepressants, although the evidence for this is not convincing.

Pyridoxine (vitamin B_6) is an enzyme concerned with tryptophane metabolism, from which 5HT is synthesized. Oral contraceptives are believed to reduce the availability of pyridoxine for normal tryptophane metabolism, and thus the formation of 5HT in the brain. Depression follows. This is the rationale for giving pyridoxine, particularly to depressed women who have been taking an oral contraceptive.

Disulfiram (Antabuse). When taken by mouth this drug interferes with the metabolism of alcohol and causes toxic metabolites to accumulate. If alcohol is ingested by a patient on Antabuse very unpleasant symptoms, occasionally fatal occur. Within 15 to 30 minutes there is generalized vasodilation and a fall of blood pressure. The patient becomes anxious, dizzy, and short of breath. His chest feels constricted and he fears a heart attack. Nausea, vomiting, and collapse may occur. Occasionally death has followed as a result of myocardial infarction. Peripheral neuritis is a rare toxic effect.

Side effects include gastrointestinal upsets and halitosis, acne, diminished libido, and tiredness. The dosage varies between 200 mg to 1.5 g a day. At least 48 hours should elapse between stopping the drug and taking alcohol.

Citrated calcium carbamide (Abstem) produces a similar effect to Antabuse when combined with alcohol, although of a less intense and dangerous nature. It needs to be taken twice a day, in doses of 50–100 mg.

ELECTRO-CONVULSIVE THERAPY (E.C.T.)

In 1933 von Meduna revived an old treatment and induced fits in his patients by injecting camphor. Camphor was replaced by cardiazol and picrotoxin, and in 1937 therapeutic fits were produced by passing an electric current across two electrodes placed on the head.

This bilateral method is still in use today but modified by the use of a muscle relaxant drug, such as suxamethonium chloride, and an anaesthetic drug, thiopentone. Unilateral E.C.T., the electrodes being placed over the non-dominant temporal and mastoid areas (i.e. on the right side of the head of a righthanded patient) is often preferred to the bilateral method. It has the advantage of causing less memory disturbance, although its effectiveness is probably not as great in deep depression, and more treatments are required than with the bilateral methods. The technique is as follows:

1. The patient fasts before treatment for five hours. If he is agitated he can be given 400 mg amylobarbitone sodium, or 10 mg nitrazepam one and a half hours before treatment.

2. Atropine 0.6 mg is given forty-five minutes before treatment.

3. The patient empties his bladder, takes out false teeth, and lies on the

bed. Intravenous thiopentone (0.25–0.5 g), followed by suxamethonium chloride (30–50 mg) is injected. A rubber gag is then inserted between the teeth.

4. After the patient has been oxygenated for a minute or so, a small current of between 90 and 150 V is passed for up to one second across padded electrodes soaked in a conducting solution. It is essential to make sure that the patient has a full fit. Signs may be almost abolished by the muscle relaxant, but flickering of the eyelids or toes can usually be seen. If the patient does not have a fit another attempt should be made at once.

5. When the fit is ended the mouth gag is removed, an airway is inserted and artificial respiration with oxygen through a B.L.B. mask is given until natural respiration restarts.

6. The patient begins to recover consciousness within a few minutes. He is at first confused and it helps if a familiar nurse can be with him at this time. Some patients become agitated during this period of confusion. This can be overcome by giving the patient an injection of diazepam or haloperidol immediately after the fit, so that he sleeps for an hour or so and wakes up relaxed with a clear mind. Usually two E.C.T. a week are given, but more can be given if necessary. There is no 'set course' of E.C.T. and the patient's progress should be assessed before each treatment. Between 4 and 12 E.C.T.'s in all may be needed for depression.

E.C.T. is a relatively safe treatment. Cardiac failure, a recent coronary thrombosis, a past history of subarachnoid haemorrhage and serious chest disease increase the possible risks.

The mode of action of E.C.T. is not known. Memory disturbances are not related to the therapeutic response, but are related to the amount of current passed. This is now minimized by using the new pulse wave machine.

MAIN INDICATIONS

(1) *Depressive illness*, particularly of the endogenous type, when it is combined with anti-depressant drugs.

(2) *Schizophrenia*. E.C.T. is given in combination with phenothiazine drugs.

(3) E.C.T. is still occasionally given for mania.

Treatment can be given on an out-patient basis. Patients are kept in the clinic after treatment until they have recovered, usually after about two hours, and then sent home in the care of a relative.

BEHAVIOUR THERAPY

Behaviour therapy covers several forms of treatment, all based on 'learning theory', that is, that neurotic symptoms or patterns of behaviour are learned, and can be 'unlearned' by certain methods.

Desensitization or reciprocal inhibition stems from Wolpe's observation that anxiety connected with a specific situation or event can be abolished by the simultaneous arousal of pleasurable feelings. The technique of desensitization depends upon teaching the patient to relax progressively until he can face the feared situation, in reality or imagination, without anxiety. A 'hierarchy' of situations is constructed, going from minimal to most frightening situations. In the case of a patient with flying phobia for instance, the minimal stimulus was to imagine the flight 6 months away, the maximum for the patient to see himself flying in a storm. With the patient relaxed and at ease, he visualizes the situation least likely to arouse anxiety. When he can do this without fear, he moves on to visualize the next situation and so on. The treatment, which is most successful in monophobias, can be carried out by nurses trained in the technique.

Operant conditioning is a useful adjunct to desensitization. The phobic patient is praised and rewarded when he completes a feared task, which thereby becomes increasingly easy.

Flooding (implosion) is in direct contrast to desensitization. Instead of teaching the patient to relax as he gradually enters the feared situation, in flooding treatment the patient immediately encounters the most frightening phobic situation he can be encouraged to endure, and has to remain with it for an hour or more until anxiety subsides. After a few sessions the patient no longer feels anxiety in the situation. It as as though he has become satiated with anxiety for that situation. Exam phobias have been dealt with most successfully by flooding techniques.

Modelling (or imitation). By imitating the therapist whom he trusts and likes, a patient is able to overcome his anxiety sufficiently to enter the phobic situation. Modelling is useful in combination with other therapies.

Atropetic therapy is a new term used to described the treatment of compulsive rituals. The patient is prevented from carrying out his rituals. This requires continual supervision for one or more weeks by the nursing staff. Physical restraint is only used as a last resort, and discussion, encouragement and persuasion are usually enough. Supervision is gradually diminished as compulsive rituals diminish.

Aversion therapy consists of associating a second response with the conditioned stimulus which is incompatible with the first response. For instance, an alcoholic is conditioned to vomit whenever he tastes alcohol, and a homosexual to feel pain from an electric shock when he desires men. We will briefly describe the technique of aversion therapy in alcoholism.

6 mg apomorphine is given intramuscularly. Nausea is felt after ten to fifteen minutes. One fluid ounce of gin or whisky, or beer if this is the usual drink of the patient, is drunk shortly before he is sick. While he is being sick further drinks are pressed on him.

The procedure is accompanied by *brain-washing*. The horrors and shame of alcoholism are emphasized, and the dangers of the *first* drink are repeatedly emphasized. The patient is told over and over again that he must *never* drink again and that he will always be *one* drink from damnation. Treatment is usually given each day for a week, with a break of one day in the middle.

ABREACTION AND NARCOANALYSIS

Narcoanalysis is the exploration of a patient's mind under the disinhibiting influence of an intravenous barbiturate or other relaxant drug. Amylobarbitone sodium, thiopentone, or methohexitone (Brietal) can be used. This technique is useful for quickly restoring memory or function in hysterical states. These drugs are not 'truth' drugs and do not *make* patients tell the truth. Sometimes a patient will recount pure fantasy.

Mild abreactions may occur when emotional material is uncovered.

EXCITATORY ABREACTIONS. Repressed memories may be brought into consciousness with an explosive release of anger or fear. Various methods are employed. They include intravenous sodium amytal, thiopentone, and still occasionally, the induction of mild anaesthesia by breathing ether or a mixture of carbon dioxide (30 per cent) and oxygen. The therapist whips up the patient's emotions to a climax, after which the patient collapses into an exhausted tearful state.

Abreaction was widely used during and immediately after the last war. Repressed traumatic incidents were abreacted with good therapeutic effect.

CONTINUOUS NARCOSIS

This was used a good deal after the barbiturates were introduced. Its main use was for treating agitated, restless or uncooperative patients. As more effective forms of therapy have developed, so the need for continuous narcosis has declined. However, there are still occasions when a modified form of continuous narcosis is useful.

The aim is to keep the patient asleep for 18–20 hours a day. A combination of chlorpromazine 100–200 mg and nitrazepam 5–10 mg and, if necessary, a small dose of a barbiturate, every 4–6 hours, is usually adequate. If necessary chlordiazepoxide 100 mg intramuscularly can be given once or twice a day. Antidepressant drugs are also given concomitantly if appropriate, and combined with E.C.T.

The drugs should be given so as to ensure the patient will be least drowsy at meal times. Fluid intake and output must be carefully watched. A minimum of two litres of fluid a day should be drunk. Apart from turning the patient every two hours or so, when possible the patient should be got out of bed at least twice a day and walked to the lavatory. This will help to avoid pulmonary and venous complications. If E.C.T. is given in conjunction the narcosis should be lighter. Continuous narcosis usually lasts between one and two weeks. Intravenous high-potency vitamins should be given regularly. Drugs should be slowly reduced over several days to avoid withdrawal effects.

MODIFIED INSULIN THERAPY

Psychiatrically ill patients frequently lose weight, particularly those with depressive or schizophrenic illness. Severe weight loss itself reduces mental stability. In fact breakdowns are not uncommon in predisposed individuals who diet excessively. It is essential therefore, when treating psychiatric patients, to ensure that lost weight is regained. But restoration of weight may be difficult when patients refuse to eat. An effective means of overcoming this difficulty is to give modified insulin treatment. This increases appetite and, because of unpleasant hypoglycaemic symptoms, to some extent forces the patient to eat.

TECHNIQUE. 10 units of soluble insulin are given at a convenient time, usually 7 a.m., to the patient in bed. This dose is increased by 10 units daily until the patient starts to sweat and shows other signs of hypoglycaemia. The average dose at which this occurs is between 30 and 60 units. An hour and a half after the injection of insulin (or before if signs of hypoglycaemia develop) the patient eats a large breakfast containing adequate amounts of carbohydrate. If hypoglycaemia develops rapidly the patient should be sat up and given a glucose drink. If this is impossible hypoglycaemia can be interrupted, either by giving a nasal feed of glucose, or by injecting glucose intravenously. In an emergency 1 mg of glucagon given intramuscularly arouses the patient within ten minutes. He must then be fed immediately. After severe hypoglycaemia the next day's dose of insulin should be halved.

After breakfast the patient gets up. He is encouraged to eat well for the rest of the day. If he goes out he must be able to recognize the signs of hypoglycaemia, and must carry a bottle of glucose in his pocket in case of need.

Some patients gain an average of 1 lb a day on such a regime, and become relaxed and cheerful. Chlorpromazine (see anorexia nervosa) is in general a simpler and safer method of putting on weight.

DEEP INSULIN THERAPY (D.I.T.). This was formerly the standard treatment of schizophrenia but has now been superseded by treatment with phenothiazine drugs.

NON-PHYSICAL TREATMENTS

1. HYPNOSIS. This has a limited value in psychiatry. The best results occur in conditions following an emotional upheaval. Hypnosis has also been used widely in psychosomatic conditions, particularly skin diseases and to induce relaxation and anaesthesia during childbirth and surgical procedures.

Hypnosis is induced by suggestion and it is essential that the hypnotist believes in his own powers. Not everyone can hypnotize, nor can everyone be hypnotized. It is estimated that 10 per cent of the population cannot be hypnotized, about 80 per cent can be hypnotized lightly, and only 10 per cent can be deeply hypnotized.

2. PSYCHOTHERAPY. This includes all forms of therapeutic communication between doctor and patient. In this sense all doctors and nurses practise psychotherapy with their patients.

There are different forms or 'levels' of psychotherapy.

1. *Authoritative.* The therapist helps the patient to re-organize his life and to deal with his major problems. It is essential that the therapist thoroughly understands his patient's personality and circumstances.

2. *Abreactive.* This is akin to the confessional box, the psychiatrist taking the place of the priest. The patient pours out his troubles, releasing a good deal of emotion in the process.

These two forms of psychotherapy are usually combined in some degree, and are sometimes referred to as *supportive psychotherapy.* Supportive psychotherapy is simpler and less time consuming than interpretative psychotherapy. By encouragement, reassurance and support the patient is helped to face and overcome his problems. The therapist, be he doctor or nurse, must be careful to view the patient's problems objectively, and not to see the patient as himself. The effectiveness of such treatment is directly related to the patient's trust and belief in the omniscience of his therapist.

3. *Interpretative.* The patient's symptoms and behaviour are interpreted to him in terms of his personality, background and current needs, with the object of giving him insight into and bringing about a radical change in his attitude and behaviour.

4. *Psychoanalysis* also aims to give a patient understanding of his behaviour and feelings, but treatment is more intense and prolonged. The patient 'free associates', that is, he says whatever comes into his mind. He is seen by the therapist up to five times a week. *Transference* describes the projection by a patient of his feelings, needs and wishes on to the analyst. A strong transference, which alternates between 'positive' and 'negative', develops in the patient for the analyst. The material brought up and the transference situation are used by the analyst in his interpretations.

Group psychotherapy. Individual psychotherapy is time consuming, and to overcome this problem groups of eight to ten patients are treated together. Techniques vary. The therapist may assume an authoritarian attitude to the group, lead the discussions and explain symptom formation and other problems. Or he may adopt a more passive role and encourage the members of the group to conduct their own discussions, only intervening to interpret at the appropriate moment.

A marital therapy groups consists of four or five married couples, each with marital difficulties. The group may be a closed one, the same members meeting together for anything up to two or three years at regular, usually weekly, intervals. Some groups are 'open-ended', its members changing continually.

A full account, for those interested, is given by Foulkes and Anthony.

MODIFIED PREFRONTAL LEUCOTOMY

Prefrontal leucotomy was introduced in 1935 by Moniz. The object of the operation is to interrupt connections between the frontal cortex and the limbic system, and so reduce emotional tension. The operation was at first too extensive and resulted in severe personality changes and epilepsy. Present-day operations have been greatly modified and aim only to sever the fibres in the lower medial quadrant of the frontal lobe. Stereotactic methods have greatly improved the accuracy of the operation. In well-selected cases personality changes are minimal. Intelligence is generally unaltered, as judged by intelligence tests.

INDICATIONS

1. Chronic, intractable tension and anxiety states.
2. Severe, long-standing obsessional states.
3. Depressive states which are severe, chronic or recurring and refractory to treatment.
4. Occasionally schizophrenic states, particularly those patients who are continually restless and prone to excited outbursts.
5. Miscellaneous states such as chronic pain, anorexia nervosa.

Symptoms should have lasted for *at least* five years, be disabling, and have failed to respond to any other treatment. Success or failure of the operation depends on being able to exclude all patients with inadequate or psychopathic personality traits. Aggressive and antisocial traits are liable to increase after operation.

RESULTS. Successful operation relieves tension and depression. Obsessional thoughts are less compelling and may gradually die out from lack of reinforcement. Paranoid ideas become less disturbing and no longer make life intolerable. There is usually some slight blunting of sensitivity, but whether this is noticeable will depend upon the patient's background.

Patients usually stay in hospital for about a month after operation, so that post operative inertia can be dealt with and former bad habits broken. Much depends upon the enthusiasm of the nursing staff in giving constant encouragement to the patient at this time. Improvement continues for six to twelve months after operation.

20

NURSE-PATIENT RELATIONSHIP

NURSES

There are many reasons why a person may wish to become a nurse. Medicine may be a family tradition. Perhaps her parents wanted her to be a nurse. Conversely, she may have taken up nursing mainly because her parents objected to the idea. Some girls play at 'nurses' from an early age, and probably identify themselves with their mothers as someone who 'nurses' the family. Others have a repressed curiosity about the human body which nursing satisfies. There are deep satisfactions to be derived from nursing. Nurses are held in high esteem by society. They form part of a respected group. It is gratifying to feel that a patient needs your help. It is satisfying to see patients recovering after serious illnesses as a result of good nursing.

But it is not easy to be a nurse. There is the anxiety of leaving home for the first time. Adolescent conflicts and difficulties may still be present and new relationships may be difficult to form. Anxiety is aroused by contact with suffering and death, human tragedy, excreta, sex, vulgarity and rudeness, and perhaps psychiatric illness. Contact with patients may arouse frightening sexual or hostile emotions which are difficult to control. Religious and moral beliefs may suddenly be lost. Anxiety may be so great as to interfere with the nurse's work.

Every nurse meets these problems. As a protection against excessive anxiety she must control her sympathy and feelings to some extent. She must be able to detach herself sufficiently from her patients to continue to nurse efficiently. But to be a good nurse she must also retain a reasonable degree of sensitivity and feeling for her patient. How these two requirements are met largely determines the sort of nurse she becomes. If she is too detached and suppresses all her emotions she will become a cold, efficient, impersonal nurse, often better suited to administration than to practical nursing. The converse is the nurse who tends to become too involved emotionally with her patients. To overcome her anxiety she overworks and insists on doing everything herself, even when she is in charge of the ward.

Particularly in their first year of training nurses may become tense and irritable. Some develop menstrual irregularities. A few relieve anxiety by over-eating or dieting. Anxiety may be reflected in off-duty behaviour. Excessive gaiety, drinking, smoking and sometimes promiscuity are more often than not due to inability to deal with anxiety in more satisfactory ways.

A well-disciplined ward, with its structural hierarchy, provides security and lessens anxiety for many. Many of the irritating customs and rules of nursing also serve to protect the nurse against anxiety. The uniforms tend to diminish individuality. If nurses carry out one particular task for all patients, such as taking temperatures or making beds, rather than attend fully to one patient, this may lessen the chance of emotional involvement with any one patient.

PATIENTS

Illness and death inevitably arouse fears and feelings of insecurity. And what frightens also fascinates. This is reflected in broadcasting, books and newspapers. Anxious people are liable to become irrational. They may deny they are ill, ignore symptoms until disease is advanced, or refuse to enter hospital. But once in a hospital bed they may change completely and become childishly dependent upon the medical staff.

Anxious people also tend to distort and exaggerate what they hear. It is important for nurses and doctors to explain fully to each patient about his illness and treatment. Although there are instances when it is better not to tell the patient everything, in general ignorance only increases a patient's anxiety.

Some patients regard all illness as a sign of weakness. They may feel they are bad and liable to earn the disapproval of society. Consequently they may be resentful and hostile to those trying to help them, and nurses need to exert considerable self-control in trying to understand them. Hostility on the part of the nurse only serves to confirm the patient's fears.

Sometimes the patient's anxiety is related to his work or his family. He may have a one-man business and face ruin as a result of a long spell of hospital treatment. Or the mother of a young family may have no one to take her place while in hospital. Less often, patients welcome the idea of entering hospital. These are usually lonely old people, to whom the security, warmth and friendship of the ward appeals.

Special problems arise with children and old people. A child may be terrified at leaving home, even when old enough to be given an explanation. His mother may be as anxious as he. In consequence she annoys the nurses by her questions or demands. Provided the nurses remain sympathetic and tolerant she will gradually become more reasonable and trusting.

Old people may be unable to adapt to the change of coming into hospital.

They become confused and disorientated, particularly at night, and develop paranoid ideas (see p. 104). Some old people value their independence as highly as life itself. They fear that hospital is the first step towards being put into an institution, and they are suspicious and resentful of the hospital staff.

Regression may occur. Behaviour becomes childlike. There may be tempers and scenes, refusal to co-operate, or alternatively a childlike dependence on the nurses. As with children, affection and reassurance are sought. Generally, the more ill the patient the greater the degree of regression. Most children regress to some extent. A boy previously dry at night may now wet the bed nightly. A child who fed himself easily may refuse to eat unless spoonfed by his nurse.

Patients come to rely on their nurses for emotional as well as physical help and comfort. A nurse may be transformed, through the patient's eyes, into a motherlike figure. She then arouses all the childhood feelings and memories of his mother in the patient. He may 'fall in love with her'. Or he may feel hostility mixed with attraction. This recreation of childish emotional feelings is known as *transference*.

Transference may occur with either sex and in varying intensity. Difficulties may be created by a patient developing such feelings for a nurse, particularly if the nurse is herself attracted to the patient. Transference situations may occur in the opposite direction, from nurse to patient. Such a situation can be very dangerous emotionally. This is one of the reasons why deeper relationships between nurses and patients are discouraged.

RECOVERY AND CONVALESCENCE

As the patient recovers his feelings of dependence fade. Sometimes a 'positive transference' may give way to negative hostile feelings. The patient for whom you have done so much may leave hospital without a word of thanks.

Most patients are very ready to leave hospital. But lonely old people, who may have little to go back to, may cling to their symptoms. Encouragement and help from a sympathetic nurse or doctor can sometimes work miracles. Symptoms from which the patient gains something may persist despite adequate treatment, and should be viewed sympathetically by the medical staff. It is unforgivable to denigrate a patient, whether deliberately or from stupidity.

PSYCHIATRIC NURSING

That psychiatric nursing differs widely from other branches of the profession is a commonly held view, especially by psychiatric nurses themselves. This is not altogether so. It is different only in so far as the *main* object of

196

effort is directed towards care of the mentally ill as opposed to caring for the physically ill, and that the nurse is required to develop a fuller, special understanding and relationship with her patients.

Before examining more closely what the psychiatric nurse actually does, it is relevant to mention here that there are two major factors which, because they affect the actual role of the nurse and other people's attitude towards her, are becoming of increasing importance.

The first is that the work of the psychiatric nurse is no longer confined to the hospital environment. Slowly, along with the established district nurse and health visitor, she is taking her place in the community as a specialist in her own right.

The second factor stems from the realization that nursing in any field involves the care of the whole person, and that patients who are hospitalized need some psychological as well as physical care. As a result, all nurses now receive some instruction in psychiatric nursing during their basic training.

Attitudes do not change overnight. There are still many people who regard mental illness as a frightening, hopeless phenomenon. They see the mentally ill as violent and dangerous, unreasonable and unreasoning, and therefore unacceptable to society, to be kept behind locked doors. In fact (except in special institutions like Broadmoor), the locked door is now the exception rather than the rule. If it is used at all, it is usually to prevent the elderly, confused patient from wandering away.

Patients' symptoms are no longer simply tolerated and contained, which was the old custodial approach. Nursing care now depends on understanding the reasons for a patient's behaviour and reacting to him in the light of such understanding. Nurses have to learn to meet the patient on equal terms, to be a person as well as a nurse to him. Some hospitals have abandoned uniforms for this reason, believing that it is not the nurse's outward appearance but her attitude which matters.

It is a stimulating, challenging time of change for nurses. Most of them are unaccustomed to being questioned at a personal level. Like doctors, they have tended to enjoy the privilege of trust in their near infallibility. Alas! This is fast disappearing in all fields of nursing, but particularly in psychiatry. Not only must the psychiatric nurse be willing to be challenged as an individual, but she must actually encourage such confrontation. In this way, the psychiatric nurse's role is very different, and she is subject to much greater stress than a nurse working in other fields.

Because every nurse is an individual, her own personal contribution to each patient's treatment programme contains something unique. Although she works according to guidelines indicated by medical staff, she has the opportunity to use her own skills and talents. Once she has developed insight into her own emotions and behaviour, she is in a position to broaden this understanding and extend it to her patients.

An important aspect of psychiatric nursing care is consistency of approach. To achieve this a nurse must understand her reactions to each patient. One way to achieve this is to discuss her feelings with a more experienced member of the treatment team, in a staff group discussion. As her confidence grows she will be able to talk with the patient himself about the feelings he has aroused in her. A remark, 'You make me feel angry when you do that', can set off a discussion which will result in increased understanding for both nurse and patient.

Psychiatric nurses in a ward may appear to an outsider to be doing little. But in fact they are intensely busy. A game of Scrabble is started by one nurse to activate a retarded depressed patient, or to make contact with a withdrawn schizophrenic, or to show her friendliness to a paranoid patient. Scrabble is a slow moving game, so that during it the nurse can observe the behaviour of other patients, not simply the one she is with, in an unobtrusive way. Later, she relays her observations to other staff members, doctors, nurses and occupational therapists, for it is important that all information is shared.

WARD AND GROUP MEETINGS.   In most psychiatric units it is now usual for patients to decide and enforce the rules necessary to control their own small and specialized community. Ward meetings of staff and patients are frequently held to discuss the daily problems that arise. Patients are encouraged to feel responsible for their own behaviour and that of their fellows. If the community as a whole has decided on a particular rule, which one patient ignores, it is more likely to be the other patients who take him to task rather than a staff member. In some therapeutic community settings the group elects a weekly chairman, who may be patient or staff. Topics for discussion include such things as how facilities can be improved or meal services speeded up, staff attitudes, why one patient always tries to dominate the meeting, why another patient resents a particular staff member or patient, or how occupational therapy can be made more interesting.

Both new patients and student nurses often feel too shy at first to speak at group meetings; the nurses particularly are conscious of their inexperience and lack of knowledge. It requires confidence to question the view of a doctor or other senior staff member and this can only be gained if the student nurses are made to feel that their observations and ideas are useful.

WARD ROUTINE.   The principles of psychiatric nursing are essentially the same whether they are practised in a short-stay unit of a general hospital, an admission ward of a psychiatric hospital, a long-stay rehabilitation ward or a psychogeriatric ward, but the routine may vary considerably.

Each ward is run according to the needs of its patients. In a *psychogeriatric* ward the routine is geared to the patients' physical as well as psychological needs. Elderly patients need a safe, homely environment where the pace is relaxed but the atmosphere still stimulating. Confused, disorientated patients require a simple ordered ward routine with opportunity for as much activity as they are capable, and some entertainment. It is important that the elderly are kept in touch with the outside world, even though they may be destined to spend their last days in hospital; television, radio and daily newspapers thus play an important part. So do visitors, and outings to the family from hospital. Many elderly patients go home regularly for weekends. Relatives can cope with them for short periods. Hospital through the week and home at the weekend is often a reasonable compromise for both.

In a *rehabilitation ward* many of the patients leave the ward each day to attend occupational or industrial therapy units, sheltered workshops or employment in a nearby town. The nurse rouses her patients early and encourages them to make their beds, and perhaps gets them to help prepare breakfast. She reminds a patient starting work for the first time to make himself a sandwich lunch, persuades another patient to have a haircut in readiness for an interview, encourages a third one to smarten himself up. She may then accompany some patients to occupational therapy and work alongside them, observing how they react to this new department. In the evening she discusses the day's work and its problems.

On an *admission* ward there are new patients for the nurse to meet, most of whom have never been in a psychiatric unit or hospital before. Many people still have preconceived ideas that psychiatric wards are horrific and patients and relatives may both need to be reassured that this is no longer so.

The way in which the admission procedure is carried out is particularly important, as first impressions are lasting. All formalities should be completed with as little fuss as possible. If the patient is reluctant to provide the nurse with the necessary information about himself he should not be pressed. This can be obtained later when he is more settled. The nurse should tell the patient what is going to happen, such as a routine physical examination, and give him general information about the time of meals, location of the bathroom and any ward rules which he will be expected to obey. Since the patient is an unknown quantity at first, he should be kept under strict observation. Observations in the acute stage of the patient's illness are, in any case, often of great diagnostic value to the doctor.

It is a good idea to introduce new patients to one or two others who have already settled in, as new patients are often mistrustful of staff at first. In this way no pressure is brought to bear on the patient, and the nurse has an opportunity to see how he reacts to other people. To force a new patient into long discussions about himself, or to make him join in group activities immediately, gives him no time to adapt to his new surroundings.

As well as receiving new patients the nurse on an admission unit is also looking after patients in various stages of treatment.

Some admission wards are often also called *observation* wards, mainly because observation and the reporting of these observations, constitutes the main work of the psychiatric nurses working in these types of units.

COMMUNITY (DOMICILARY) PSYCHIATRIC NURSING. In addition to the well-established out-patient system, this service is now being supplemented in many areas by a community psychiatric nursing service. As well as attending hospital for a follow-up out-patient appointment with his doctor, the patient is also visited regularly in his home by an experienced psychiatric nurse.

This is an extremely valuable development for both patients and nurses alike. Often, it is impossible for the hospital doctor or nurse to gain a clear picture of the home environment of their patient. The psychiatric social worker takes a history from the patient and his relatives concerning the family circumstances, but this may merely represent the picture they wish to present. First-hand impressions gained by a visiting nurse can be far more enlightening.

It is easier to judge a person in the setting of his home than in hospital. Relationships between the patient and other family members soon become clear, particularly as they come to accept the nurse's presence. The community psychiatric nurse who visits a patient after discharge often learns more about the psychodynamics underlying his symptoms and difficulties than the hospital staff were ever able to do. Armed with this knowledge the nurse is strongly placed to prevent relapse and readmission to hospital. She is in a position to assess the extent of his recovery and what further treatment he may need.

One of the most important advantages of a community psychiatric nursing service is that it provides the vital link with hospital which a patient so often needs after his discharge. Many patients are frightened and sometimes openly reluctant to be discharged, apprehensive at the thought of having no doctor or nurse on hand. Psychiatric nurses sometimes receive invitations to visit a patient's home. Usually these invitations are extended under the guise of gratitude for what the nurse has done for the patient. In reality, of course, what the patient is really saying is that he is frightened to leave the safe hospital environment.

As a general rule, invitations of this kind are best refused. An inexperienced nurse may find herself in the uncomfortable position of being unable to withdraw from the situation without appearing rude and rejecting. Nurses are wise to remember that a patient may need readmission. Once the professional relationship has become a more personal one it may be impossible to re-establish it on a purely professional basis. In addition, patients who develop a friendship with their nurse are liable to become over-intense and demanding. It will therefore ultimately prove unsatisfactory for both people. It is better for the nurse to reverse the invitation and ask him back to the hospital. For this reason social evenings are often regularly organized and many hospitals have flourishing clubs run by discharged patients and interested staff members.

COMMUNITY CARE

An adequate community care system, able to provide supervision, day hospitals, hostels and sheltered workshops for discharged patients is essential is psychiatric units in general hospitals are to replace the mental hospitals Local authorities should (but are not obliged to) set up various facilities.

1. *Hostels and sheltered residential accommodation.* A period of residence in a *half-way house* or hostel may help the patient who is discharged after a long-time in hospital to adjust to the responsibilities of everyday life before emerging fully into the community. He is able to go out to work, knowing that his general needs will be looked after. Residential accommodation is also needed for elderly patients who are not capable of living alone or in small families, but who do not yet need care in hospital. Hostel accommodation may also be required for mentally subnormal children whose homes are situated a long way from a training centre.

Residential accommodation is also provided by the Mental After-Care Association.

2. *Therapeutic social clubs and centres*, which help to offset the bad effects of loneliness.

3. *Day Centres and Day Hospitals. Night Hospitals.*

Patients not needing or unwilling to accept complete hospitalization, but requiring more intensive treatment than an ordinary out-patient clinic can provide, benefit from treatment in a day hospital. Day hospitals cater ideally for between 20 and 30 patients at a time, attending five days a week between 9 a.m. to 4 p.m. All forms of treatment are given, and all types of patient treated there. Group therapy is particularly useful in such a setting. Close co-operation is required between nurses, occupational therapists and doctors. Recently, as in the *Worthing Scheme*, early treatment in a day hospital has reduced the admission rate of patients to the parent hospital. Day centres are particularly useful for elderly patients who cannot be left alone, or whose relatives need a respite from them.

Patients who are capable of working, but are too disturbed for ordinary family life, often improve slowly if they can continue to work. This is sometimes possible in the absence of a halfway house, by arranging for them to return from work to a *night hospital*.

4. *The Disablement Resettlement Service* helps registered disabled persons to obtain and keep suitable work. All employers of twenty or more people must employ a quota of disabled people, and certain jobs such as lift and car park attendants are reserved for them. A *disablement resettlement officer* (D.R.O.) is attached to each labour exchange. He will help in one of four ways:

(a) Find a suitable job.

(b) For people fit only for *sheltered* employment, special facilities exist with non-profit making firms, such as Remploy Ltd. Such protected work is essential for the partially recovered schizophrenic.

(c) He may arrange for the person to go to an *Industrial Rehabilitation Unit*. There he will be gradually reconditioned to the stresses of industrial life.

(d) He may arrange *vocational training* at a Government training centre.

(N.B.—There are 800 000 registered disabled people, of whom 74 000 have psychiatric disorders.)

5. Many more skilled workers are required to supervise and help the patient and his family. More *psychiatric social workers*, *health visitors*, nurses with psychiatric training and other ancillary workers are needed if the community care system is to be effective.

It must also be realized that the *general practitioner* plays a vital part in the community care services. He is the person best placed to diagnose and deal with early psychiatric disease. And all too often the whole brunt of looking after discharged psychiatric patients falls on him.

21

MEDICO-LEGAL

THE COMPULSORY ADMISSION OF PATIENTS TO HOSPITAL

MENTAL HEALTH ACT OF 1959. Until the *Mental Treatment Act of 1930*, allowing for voluntary admission, patients requiring admission to mental hospitals had to be certified insane. By the 1950s, although most admissions were voluntary, the ancient laws were proving increasingly inadequate. Accordingly, in 1954 the Government set up a Royal Commission on 'the Law relating to Mental Illness and Mental Deficiency', which resulted in the 1959 *Mental Health Act*.

The Mental Health Act of 1959 broke the artificial legal barrier that separated psychiatry from the rest of medicine. A patient suffering from a mental illness is now entitled to receive the same facilities for treatment as any other type of patient, and to enter any hospital without legal formality.

The term *mental disorder* is used in a wide sense to mean mental illness, arrested or incomplete development of mind, psychopathic disorder, and any other disorder or disability of mind.

Although the vast majority of admissions are informal, *compulsory admission* is still needed on occasion. A patient may be so disturbed as to need to be detained 'in the interests of his own health or safety or with a view to the protection of other persons.' An application on a special form accompanied by the recommendations of two medical practitioners, is made by the nearest relative *or* mental welfare officer to the medical superintendent of the hospital to which admission is sought. One of the practitioners must be a psychiatric specialist, approved for the purpose by the local health authority. The other should preferably be the patient's general practitioner. Under Section 25 a patient may be admitted for observation and compulsorily detained for not more than 28 days. Under Section 26, a patient may be detained for treatment for up to a year.

In an emergency (Section 29) a patient can be admitted on the strength of one medical recommendation. A second medical recommendation must reach the medical superintendent of the hospital within 72 hours, otherwise the application automatically expires.

Normally the consultant looking after the detained patient decides

203

when he is fit for discharge. But the detained patient, or his nearest relative has the right to apply to a *Mental Health Review Tribunal* for discharge within six months of his admission. The Tribunal consists of at least three people, including a lawyer, doctor and a layman with knowledge of the social services. Their decision concerning continued detention or discharge is final.

A patient can be detained for *observation* (Section 25) for up to 28 days. At the end of this time, if compulsion is still necessary, he can be detained for treatment. Patients can be detained *for treatment* (Section 26) in hospital for one year. At the end of this time the detention order can be extended for a further year, and subsequently for two one-year periods. The patient and his relatives may appeal to the Mental Health Review Tribunal after each renewal.

(For compulsory detention of a psychopath see p. 204).

GUARDIANSHIP

Special legal procedures exist for boarding out certain patients who are subnormal or mentally ill, known as guardianship.

TESTAMENTARY CAPACITY

The validity of a will depends on the mental state of the person concerned at the time. He may be mentally ill but still be capable of making a will, provided that he knows (a) the extent and nature of his possessions, (b) those who might expect to benefit and (c) his judgement is not clouded or warped.

Appendix
DRUGS IN COMMON USE

Amphetamines still in common use include

Dexamphetamine (Dexedrine)
Drinamyl (Amphetamine combined with Amytal)
Steladex (Amphetamine combined with stelazine)
Other stimulants include
Methylphenidate (Ritalin)
Phenmetrazine (Preludin)
Fenfluramine (Ponderax)
Pemoline (Kethamid)
All the drugs produced to suppress appetite probably have more or less of a stimulating effect depending on the patient's personality.

ANTIDEPRESSANT DRUGS

Monoamine oxidase inhibitors

Iproniazid (Marsilid)
Phenelzine (Nardil)
Isocarboxazid (Marplan)
Mebanazine (Actomol)
Nialamide (Niamid)
Tranylcypromine (Parnate)

Tricyclic compounds

Imipramine (Tofranil)
Amitriptyline (Tryptizol, Saroten)
Nortriptyline (Aventyl, Allegron)
Trimipramine (Surmontil)
Protriptyline (Concordin)
Iprindole (Prondol)
Desimpramine (Petrofran)
Clomipramine (Anafranil)
Doxepin (Sinequan)
Dothiepin (Prothiaden)
Dibenzepin (Noveril)

TRANQUILLIZER DRUGS

Major tranquillizers

(*a*) *Phenothiazine derivatives*
Chlorpromazine (Largactil)
Thioridazine (Melleril)
Trifluoperazine (Stelazine)
Perphenazine (Fentazin)
Fluphenazine (Moditen)
Long-acting fluphenazine preparations (Moditen and Modecate)

(*b*) *Butyrophenone derivatives*
Haloperidol (Serenace)
Trifluoperidol (Triperidol)

(*c*) Oxypertine (Integrin)
Pimozide (Orap)

Minor tranquillizers

(*d*) *Diazepine derivatives:*
Chlorodiazepoxide (Librium)
Diazepam (Valium)
Medazepam (Nobrium)
Oxazepam (Serenid)
Potassium chlorazepate (Tranxene)
(*b*) Meprobamate (Equanil, Miltown)
(*c*) Benzoctamine (Tacitin)

HYPNOTICS

Barbiturates:

Pentobarbitone (Nembutal)
Sodium amylobarbitone (Sodium Amytal)
Quinalbarbitone (Seconal)
Butobarbitone (Soneryl)

Non-barbiturates:

Glutethimide (Doriden)
Nitrazepam (Mogadon)
Methaqualone (Mellsil)
Methaqualone and diphenhydramine (Mandrax)

Glossary

ABREACTION. Reliving past events with a release of emotion.

AMNESIA. Loss of memory.

ANIMISM. Thinking of external objects as 'alive' and having feelings similar to your own.

ANXIETY STATE. A continual and irrational feeling of anxiety in the absence of any justifiable cause.

BEHAVIOUR THERAPY. Behaviour therapy is based on the theory that neurotic symptoms or patterns of behaviour are learned, unadaptive responses to a conditioned stimulus, and they can be 'unlearned' by certain methods.

BELLE INDIFFERENCE. The unconcern shown by a hysterical patient about his symptoms.

CHARACTER. A person's qualities, attitudes and expected behaviour.

CLOUDING OF CONSCIOUSNESS. A mental state in which awareness is diminished or lost.

COMPLEX. Ideas which are emotionally unacceptable and have therefore been repressed, but continue to influence behaviour and thought.

COMPULSIVE NEUROSIS. An impulse or movement which an individual feels compelled to carry out, usually repetitively, in spite of a strong urge to resist.

CONFABULATION. A word describing the fabrication which a patient with loss of memory may employ to fill in the gaps in his memory.

CONDITIONED REFLEX. A simple reflex which has been modified so that it is now evoked by a stimulus different from the 'natural' one.

CONTINUOUS NARCOSIS. A form of treatment in which the patient is kept asleep for up to twenty hours a day.

CONVERSION. Changing a repressed wish into a bodily symptom, as occurs in hysteria.

CULTURE. The values, beliefs, accepted patterns of behaviour and customs accumulated by a society.

CYCLOTHYMIC PERSONALITY. An individual whose mood constantly fluctuates, often for little or no apparent cause, between elation and depression.

DECONDITIONING. Abolishing a conditioned reflex by applying another stimulus between the conditioned stimulus and the expected response.

DÉJÀ VU. The sense of familiarity, associated with a feeling of 'having been there before', or reliving experiences from some earlier state of existence.

DELIRIUM. A state of reversible confusion.

DELUSION. A false belief.

DEMENTIA. A state of permanent, and often progressive, intellectual impairment.

DEPERSONALIZATION. A feeling that you have changed, and the world is seen as though in a dream.

DIPSOMANIA. A form of alcoholism.

DISPLACEMENT. A mental mechanism whereby anxiety is switched from what is really feared to some apparently unconnected object or situation.

DISSOCIATION. A mental mechanism which results in 'splitting of consciousness' so that inconsistencies in thought or behaviour are overlooked.

EGO. A psychoanalytical term for the conscious part of the mind.

EGOCENTRIC THOUGHT. Thought which is controlled more by inner needs and wishes than by reality. It is typical of young children.

EIDETIC IMAGERY. A very vivid form of visual imagery, in which past scenes are reproduced with almost photographic accuracy and clearness.

EMOTION. A subjective feeling combined with certain bodily changes.

EXTRAVERT. A sociable, outgoing person.

FUGUE. Loss of memory in a patient who has 'wandered' off from home.

GROUP PSYCHOTHERAPY. A form of treatment in which groups of patients discuss one another's problems, as well as their own.

HALLUCINATION. Percepts that occur in the absence of any external stimuli. They cannot therefore be perceived by other people.

HETEROSEXUALITY. Sexual attraction for someone of the opposite sex.

HOMEOSTASIS. Maintaining the 'internal environment' of the body.

HOMOSEXUALITY. Sexual attraction for someone of the same sex.

HYPNOGOGIC HALLUCINATION. Hallucinations experienced at the moment of dropping off or awakening from sleep.

HYPOCHONDRIASIS. Preoccupation with bodily functions and sensations.

HYSTERIA. A disorder in which physical symptoms or certain mental disturbances occur in the absence of organic disease.

HYSTERICAL PERSONALITY. An emotionally shallow, selfish, demanding person.

IDEAS OF REFERENCE. Delusional beliefs that certain external events are especially related to the individual.

IDENTIFICATION. Imitating an admired person.

ILLUSION. An error of perception whereby stimuli are wrongly interpreted.

IMAGERY. The process of seeing with the mind's eye' something that is not actually real or present at the time.

INSTINCT. Unlearned, inherited patterns of behaviour.

INTELLIGENCE. The ability to reason and to think rationally and purposefully.

INTELLIGENCE QUOTIENT (I.Q.). The ratio of mental age over chronological age × 100.

INTROVERT. A reserved, rather unsociable type of person.

MANIA. A condition characterized by elation and overactivity.

MEMORY. A mental process consisting of registering, retaining, recalling and recognizing 'information'.

MENTAL AGE. The age at which the 'average' child would have passed the intelligence tests the individual concerned has passed.

MENTAL DEFECT. This term has now been replaced by subnormality.

NEURASTHENIA. A state of inexplicable fatigue.

NEUROSIS. A condition in which the patient recognizes that he is mentally ill.

OBSESSIONAL NEUROSIS. An obsession is a thought, impulse or movement which an individual feels compelled to carry out, usually repetitively, in spite of a strong urge to resist.

OBSESSIONAL PERSONALITY. Someone who tends to be over-conscientious and self-exacting.

OCCUPATIONAL THERAPY. Therapeutic work.

OMNIPOTENCE. Feeling of tremendous power.

PARAPHRENIA. A form of schizophrenia starting relatively late in life, where the personality is well preserved.

PERCEPTION. The process of selection and organization of stimuli by the brain whereby we become aware of what is happening around and in our bodies.

PERSONALITY. This is the *whole* person, his attitudes, moods, characteristic behaviour, the way he parts his hair, the type of girl friend he has, the books he likes, his height, and so on.

PHANTASY. Undirected, uncontrolled thought.

PHOBIA. A specific fear of something.

PREJUDICE. Fixed beliefs which are unfavourable to the objects concerned.

PRESENILE DEMENTIA. Dementia occuring usually between the ages of forty and sixty.

PROJECTION. Displacing unacceptable attitudes and feelings on to someone else.

PSYCHIATRY. The study and treatment of disordered mental processes.

PSYCHOANALYSIS. A form of treatment in which unconscious memories are brought to light by 'free association', by allowing thoughts to wander without conscious direction.

PSYCHOLOGY. The study and understanding of normal mental functions and behaviour.

PSYCHOPATH. An individual who has little or no sense of right and wrong.

PSYCHOPATHOLOGY. The past events in a patient's life which may have contributed to his present illness.

PSYCHOSIS. An illness in which the patient does not recognize that he is ill and his whole personality is involved in and changed by the illness.

PSYCHOSOMATIC. Physical conditions or symptoms for which emotional factors are responsible, or in which they play a major role.

PSYCHOTHERAPY. Treatment depending on therapeutic communication between doctor and patient.

REACTION FORMATION. A mental mechanism by which unconscious wishes result in the opposite attitudes and behaviour being adopted consciously.

REASONING. Thought controlled and directed purposefully.

REFLEX (SIMPLE). An inborn, involuntary, automatic response to a stimulus.

REGRESSION. Returning to earlier, more childish, forms of behaviour.

REPRESSION. The involuntary process by which ideas unacceptable to the conscience, or super-ego, are pushed out of consciousness.

SCHIZOID PERSONALITY. A solitary individual lacking emotional warmth.

STEREOTYPE. Groups of fixed, oversimplified and generalized conceptions. When these conceptions are unfavourably they are linked with prejudice.

SUBLIMATION. Directing undesirable tendencies into socially acceptable channels.

SUPER EGO. Psychoanalytical term for conscience.

TEMPERAMENT. The characteristic mood of an individual.

THOUGHT. Conscious mental activity.

THOUGHT BLOCKING. Interference with the 'normal' train of thought; it occurs in schizophrenia.

TRANSFERENCE. A term used to describe the dependent and often childlike relationship which sometimes forms between patients and medical staff.

UNREALITY. A feeling that the world, rather than you, has 'changed', and become colourless and meaningless.

Books Recommended for Reading

ACKERKNECHT, E. H. *A Short History of Psychiatry*. 1959. Hasner Publishing Company, New York.

ARTHUR, J. R. *Introduction to Social Psychiatry*. 1971. Penguin Books, London.

BOWLBY, J. *Attachment and Loss, Vol.* 1. 1969. Hogarth Press, London.

BROWN, J. A. C. *The Social Psychology of Industry*. 1958. Penguin Books, London.

DALLY, P. *Anorexia Nervosa*. 1969. Heinemann Medical Books, London.

DALLY, P. *Chemotherapy of Psychiatric Disorders*. 1967. Logos Press, London.

DAVIS, D. R. *An Introduction to Psychopathology*. 1957. Oxford University Press, London.

ELKIN, F. *The Child and Society*. 1961. Random House, New York.

EYSENCK, H. J. *Know Your Own I.Q.*. 1962. Penguin Books, London.

FERARD, L. N. and HUNNYBUN, K. *The Caseworker's Use of Relationships*. 1962. Tavistock Publications, London.

FOULKES, S. H. and ANTHONY, E. J. *Group Psychotherapy*, 1957. Penguin Books, London.

FREUD, S. *The Interpretation of Dreams*. 1953. Hogarth Press, London.

GRINKER, R. R. *Psychosomatic Research*. 1961. Grove Press, New York.

HART. B. *The Psychology of Insanity*. 1962. Cambridge University Press.

HUNTER, I. M. L. *Memory*. 1961. Penguin Books, London.

LAING, R. D. and ESTERSON, A. *Sanity, Madness and The Family*. Tavistock Publications, 1964. London.

LORENZ, K. Z. *King Solomon's Ring*. 1961. University Paperbacks. Methuen. London.

MAIRET, P. *Christian Essays in Psychiatry*. 1956, S.C.M. Press Ltd. London.

MITTLER, P. *The Study of Twins*. 1971. Penguin Books, London.

SARGANT, W. *Battle for the Mind*. Heinemann 1960.

STORR, A. *The Integrity of the Personality*. 1963. Penguin Books, London.

STORR, A. *Sexual Deviation*. 1964. Penguin Books, London.

THOMPSON, R. *The Psychology of Thinking*. 1959. Penguin Books, London.

WOLFF, S. *Children under Stress*. 1969. Allen Lane, The Penguin Press, London.

Index